To Stacey
and for all
those who follow —

Fondly

Bev Bryant

TO

WHEREVER

OCEANS

GO

By Beverley Bryant

Published by **Wings**
South Paris, Maine

Published by

WINGS

South Paris, Maine

Copyright c 1996 by Beverley Bryant
All Rights Reserved

No part of this book may be reproduced in any form or transmitted by any electronically or mechanical means, including photocopying, recording or by any information storage and retrieval systems, without permission in writing from the author. Exceptions will be granted for reviewers who may quote brief passages for reviews in newspapers, other periodicals and broadcasts. Written requests for permission are welcomed to be sent to Beverley Bryant, 1 Clifford Court, South Paris, Maine 04281 or call 207-743-8173.

First Edition 1996

ISBN 1 882332-01-6

DEDICATION
TO

Rita Oliverio	and	***Koko Keller***
who		who
Let me cry		Made me laugh
Never questioned		Questioned everything
Listened to my "roots"		Breathed life into "Wings"
Taught me to follow		Urged me to lead
Calmed my panic attacks		Panicked my calm attacks
Isolated the problems		Created solutions
Got me started		Brought me home
Had "ears" with a heart		Had a "heart" with ears

....during my process of becoming....
and

Marcia Cooper, *my dear friend...who laughed with me, and flew with me, and cried with me, and grew with me.. and who kept me inspired with her love.*
And to
*to **my family**, for loving who I was, who I am and who I will be.*

Table of Contents

Introduction 10

SECTION ONE: A STARTING POINT

Chapter 1   Driftwood: To Begin Again 16
Chapter 2   Before The Storm 29
Chapter 3   From Gordon's Perspective .... .38

SECTION TWO: RIDING OUT THE STORM

Chapter 4   The Awakenings 50
Chapter 5   The Turning Of The Tides 65
Chapter 6   Going Back To The Beginning 73
Chapter 7   Taking the Wheel 79
Chapter 8   From Kimberly's Perspective 83

SECTION THREE: AT THE HELM

Chapter 9   Running With The Tide 92
Chapter 10 The Last Hurrah 105
Chapter 11 The Final Straw 109

SECTION FOUR: TOWARD NEW HORIZONS

Chapter 12 The Book 122
Chapter 13 Redesigning Destinations 136

Table of Contents

SECTION FIVE: IMPRINTS

Chapter 14 From Carrie's Perspective............................148
Chapter 15 Challenges: Book 2......................................159
Chapter 16 When The Tide Changes, Go With
            The Current: Challenges From Within.......167
Chapter 17 From Mark's Perspective.............................176
Chapter 18 Building Life Rafts.......................................182

SECTION SIX: REBUILDING ME

Chapter 19 Relearning To Swim....................................199
Chapter 20 Reaching The Shore.....................................227

SECTION SEVEN: THE WEATHER TODAY-
             THE FORECAST TOMORROW

Chapter 21 Survival Techniques.....................................237
Chapter 22 In Honor Of The Crew................................250
Chapter 23 Revisiting The Beach...................................274
Chapter 24 Epilogue: The Call Of The Gulls...............284

INTRODUCTION

My book is about brain injury. But it is also about people, and how they deal with life. How we come to realize that the power to recover lies deep within each of us. We have only to realize it and call upon that strength to heal ourselves. Sustaining a brain injury leavesa person different than before, and coming to grips with the process of "becoming a person that you like" again, is a long and arduous process.

Acquired brain injury or (ABI) occurs every 15 seconds to someone in the United States of America. It hits fast, like a tsunami, and leaves lifelong devastation in its wake. Acquired brain injury changes you instantly. Injuries can be termed mild, moderate or severe, but the one thing I have learned is that recovery is long, hard and heart-wrenching in all three cases. I have lived with the remnants of brain injury and fought hard against the tides of sympathy and apathy. I know I could not endure another injury, so I take the necessary precautions now. Buckling seat belts, wearing helmets, and promoting awareness have become a part of my life.

Maybe we need to have that tidal wave hit us head on before we listen and learn. I certainly hope that is not true.

Motor vehicle accidents, falls and violence are the leading causes of ABI, which is the leading killer of children and young adults in our country today. It would be wonderful if we could all learn to love and protect each other, eliminate accidents and the growing violence. But wishing won't make it happen. The only avenue left is to make others aware of the permanency of brain injury through education.

There is no cure!....only prevention. So it is vital that people learn how to begin the healing process. Long after the physicians have gone home; long after the therapists have finished; long after the bones have mended; people who have sustained brain injury still struggle to recover and heal. Healing takes place from the inside out. Healing involves the struggle to rebuild relationships with family, friends, and colleagues. Healing is recognizing the grieving process and coming to grips with our remaining strengths, asking for accommodation, using strategies, compensating for weaknesses, and believing in ourselves.

There are many aspects of sustaining a brain injury. When you have been the one to undergo the discrimination, the insults, the hardships, the stares, the lack of understanding, the losses, then you might begin to realize the complexity of brain injury from our perspective. Acquired brain injury occurs suddenly, in one moment in time, and changes our lives immediately and yet, for the long term too. We are often misdiagnosed, and unvalidated. Testing is complicated and expensive for milder head injury and often, only a neuropsychologist can identify needs and losses. In this, the decade of the brain, doctors are still struggling to learn how the brain works and the scientific world of research is just getting the technology that can enter the microscopic cellular stage of discovery on the working brain.

There is no doubt that persons who have sustained a brain injury need help, but it must be specific help that is geared to the individual. There are few rehabilitation counselors, outside of brain injury rehabilitation centers, that have any understanding of brain injury and how to deal with it in the workplace or school. We are left to seek out our own help, transitions, and solutions.

But we are changed after brain injury, and learning to live with a new "self" is, often very frustrating and exhausting. Effects quickly spread to those nearby. Some people refer to these effects as ripples. They are not ripples. They are full-blown waves that hit the family head on, and smother them with immediate and long-term problems. These problems need solutions, such as where to find help, finances, energy and time to care for their loved one, and living with the changes they find themselves facing.

These same waves overwhelm friends and, in

many cases, carry them off. They isolate the survivors, and eventually lead to bewilderment and a very questioning of their own worth. If survivors are lucky enough to have a job and be able to go back to work, these waves often alienate colleagues, leaving the survivor ineffective and vulnerable and not understanding why.

Learning to return to work is a long, complicated process that needs genuine caring and nurturing. The sequelae of brain injury keep washing away the castles that one struggles to build in the remaining sand. Survivors are left in an undertow, that is always there with the outgoing tide: An undertow that is constantly pulling the survivors and their families under, and deluging them with problems that seem to have no solution. It is with these waves that this book concerns itself and tries to offer help, understanding and encouragement.

ABI affects everyone around us, changing family, friends, colleagues, and even strangers. When the initial impact is over and the tide recedes, no one is ever the same again.

With my vast cognitive deficits, I sometimes feel that I have wandered among the Alzheimers's ward as a patient, and somehow, have been privileged to return to a world they can't. That makes me feel very special, often as though there is a reason for my experience. We all search for reasons, to make experiences meaningful. I hope all who read this come to know the importance of trying to look at the world through the perspective of those who have lived it, and try to see it through their eyes.

My first book, IN SEARCH OF WINGS, tells of my struggles through the early rehabilitative experience, so I won't dwell on that part of the journey here. One part effects the other, so we sometimes need to go back there, in order to understand the present. This story begins in a new place, further on in my journey, beyond the curing. It begins at the "healing wall", a wall where we begin to discover ourselves again, find an inner worth to guide us, live each day for all its worth, and begin to realize that there are no limits to the human potential. There never were.

SECTION ONE

A STARTING POINT

CHAPTER ONE

"DRIFTWOOD"

...To Begin Again...

It is a very dark night and I still have a couple of errands to do before heading homeward. As I drive slowly toward the turnpike toll booth, carefully taking a quarter from my change tray between the seats, I feel a rush of excitement.

I used to have problems deciding what lane to get into, as traffic merged from many lanes down to a few. But now my mind is racing ahead, trying to repeat my two errands. We need bread and milk for morning, so I need to stop at the grocery store in Gray.

As I approach the toll booth, I notice some lanes ahead with red lights over them, and some with blinking lights. Staying in the lane I am in, I proceed straight ahead to the red light and stop my car.

As I wait patiently, I allow my mind to wander back to only two years earlier, when I had sustained traumatic brain injury in a car accident. It has been a very long two years. I have dealt with recovery from many different aspects. There have been times when I felt I would never be out of a wheelchair. There were times when I felt I would never be able to be left alone and unsupervised again. But the worst times were when I thought about the possibility of never being able to drive again. I had wanted to achieve that more than anything else, and had worked endlessly to reach that goal. Now, here I am, driving at night, alone in my car. I have come such a long, long way.

......

"The horns are blowing and I don't know why. Do they think I am going to go through this red light, for God's sake? I know enough not to do that."

......

My thoughts casually returned again to the past. There were people, some of the most respected professionals in the country, who had predicted I would never drive again. At times I found it hard not to believe them, too. But I kept my motivation and determination and laid the last bit of faith I could muster into my instincts. With much therapy and many strategies, I had come this far. If some of those people could only see me now. I felt a great deal of self-satisfaction, while my fingers continued to fondle the quarter in my hand for the toll.

As I patiently waited for the red light to turn green, the horns started to blow, and oncoming headlights exposed me to the world. Angry toll takers began gesturing me from within their lighted booths. It took a few seconds to process what was happening. Suddenly I felt the world caving in around me. I looked over to the three lanes on my right, with green lights flashing above them. They were there to let me know it was OK to pass through. I had driven into the lane with the red light. With much deliberate care, I had stopped my car without driving through, and suddenly was the focus of many irate drivers waiting to pass through from the other side.

I finally realized that this red light was never going to change to green, and I needed to make a decision fast. I think my healing began as I meekly changed lanes and moved out of the way of a very impatient "18 wheeler", coming straight at me through the toll booth from the other direction. I think I made a very good decision.

Sometimes God has his own way of keeping us humble and reminding us of our limitations. I had just been reminded that I still was a person with a brain injury.

As I handed the toll taker my quarter, he passed me a toll ticket. In my distraction, I forgot that we pay when we get off, not when we get on the turnpike. Taking the ticket sheepishly, I apologized for my forgetfulness, and put the ticket over my visor. As I picked up speed and started homeward, I tossed the quarter into my change tray. As if trying to escape my inconsistency, it bounced out of the change tray and onto the floor and rolled under my feet. I guess I had the feeling then, of things to come, before my day was over. I thought about the past.

······

My car accident had occurred during a blizzard on a back road in the western foothills of Maine. I spent long weeks in a rehabilitation hospital, and went through two years of outpatient therapy to recover some of my cognitive skills. I spent even longer learning strategies and compensational techniques to deal with the skills I had lost. I used every bit of effort and energy I had, to keep believing that I would eventually return to my former level of functioning. I tried to never let anyone see my frustration and always give my therapists and myself 110% of my effort.

Being a genuinely happy person before my accident, I tended to be very optimistic in all things. It had helped when the going got rough. Also being a gymnastics judge for twenty-four years, I had spent much of my life looking at defects in performance. My experience in analyzing faults and studying mechanical aspects of correcting them, was very helpful in dealing with my own recovery. I was able to devise new and creative ways to use strategies to help myself, but first the professionals had to tell me what was wrong. My brain injury affected my self-monitoring, awareness, reasoning, judgment, thought processing, attention, short-term memory, as well as my ability to recognize that I had any problems.

During eleven months in physical therapy, six months in occupational therapy, and over a year and a half in speech therapy, I had given them my best shot. I had been very fortunate to have good therapists who cared about me as a person: Not only as a client and patient, but as a friend as well. Many times that was what made the difference. I was able to relate to someone, have a role model or mentor, and learn, while I was experiencing my mistakes in the community with real people and in real life situations.

I, also, had a problems with initiation after my injury. Initiation is the ability to get started. My "starter button" no longer worked right. While I could understand the strategies I learned, it was very difficult to use them when I needed to. I had learned well what to do. I just simply never did it. So, having someone with me, helped to remind me, until I could initiate some action myself. This also enabled me to eventually transfer learned strategies to new and different situations as they became internalized.

I dealt with problems relating to fatigue, endurance, distractibility, attention, concentration, perseveration, focusing, over-stimulation, disinhibition and impulsivity, to name a few. Some of my deficits didn't show up until later in my recovery. Maybe they were there from the beginning, but I didn't recognize them until I found myself in more complex situations. I displayed behavioral changes in dealing with anger, confrontation, and anything emotional in nature. My husband and family were embarrassed by my actions and language. I lost control if I had to deal with changes quickly or anyone who was angry. I developed panic attacks at certain sounds, and would "run" and then become disoriented.

Because of my short-term memory loss, I would argue vehemently with anyone that something never happened, even though those I loved and respected assured me that it did. I eventually lost confidence in myself, because I was never sure if I could trust my instincts anymore. I was one who had been full of confidence before my accident. I worked in the most tense situations, where others would have died of fright, and worked with a casualness and calmness rarely seen. I couldn't understand how I could have changed so much because of a bump on the head. I did things so differently. I thought and perceived things in another light. I acted and reacted much more unpredictably now. I no longer learned by just scanning information. I now no longer learned anything.

There seemed to be two of us in one body now--the old me and the new me. At times, it was damn hard trying to live up to the expectations of either of us.

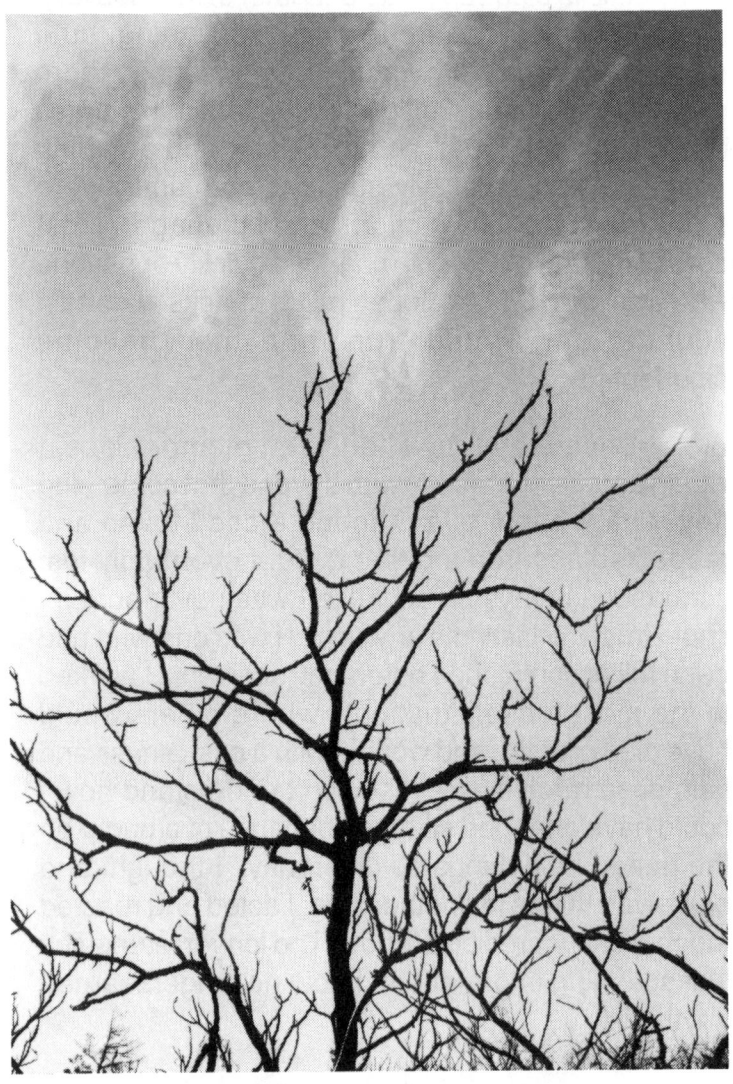

THE STRANGER WITHIN

We are like driftwood,
You and I,
Sometimes still and lifeless
A remnant of a passing catastrophe.

We are like seaweed,
You and I,
Floating on a sea of sunlight,
A sign that living things survive.

We are like black and white,
You and I,
Being pulled together in the undertow,
Fighting each other all the way down.

We are like Moses in the bulrush,
You and I,
Resting from what lies in store for us
In the puckerbrush beyond.

We are like stars in the midnight sky,
You and I,
Giving off a glow that daylight cannot diminish
Oblivious to those watching.

We are so different, yet so the same.
You and I,
Remnants of a tidal wave passing,
An eternity, in less than a moment.

Living with a brain injury is like enduring a perennial existence of "toll booth experiences". I was never sure if what I was doing was correct, acceptable, or even the desired response. Recovery from brain injury is like stepping into a world where nothing is for certain, and in time, you question the validity of even your most automatic behaviors. It is a world full of dichotomies and similarities, and it is often hard to tell the difference.

One incident that is indelibly inscribed on my patchy memory cells, serves to remind me how fragile, reality is for us. It happened about six months after I was discharged as an inpatient at the rehabilitation hospital. I was still under 24-hour supervisional care (meaning I was not allowed to be left alone). On our way home from therapy, Gordon had taken me with him to a local hardware discount superstore. He needed to shop for plumbing supplies for our apartments.

Once there, he picked up an assortment of little items and then needed to find a salesman to make arrangements to purchase a bathtub. Preferring not to take the shopping cart with him, he asked me to stay at that spot and wait for him until he returned. Very carefully and thoughtfully he rearranged some boxes on the side of the aisle, so that I could sit while I waited.

I climbed up on the boxes and watched as he disappeared. After a few minutes I became bored and restless. I had been taught strategies to take my mind off impulsive urges during my therapy. One of my favorites was to sing to myself. So I began to sing, but not to myself unfortunately. The boxes were so high that my feet couldn't touch the floor, and several men passing by, gave odd looks to this strange, middle-aged lady, totally contented, swinging her legs and singing.

All of a sudden in the middle of one of my songs, I looked up and there was Dr. Caldwell, the physiatrist (a medical doctor trained in rehabilitation) from the hospital who was in charge of my care. Knowing that I was not to be left alone because of my wandering, he looked at me and said, "Beverley, What are you doing here?" I answered very proudly that I was doing exactly what I was supposed to for a change. I told him "Gordon told me to sit here and not move one inch, and I am doing it". He asked, "Where's Gordon?". I said, "I don't know where he is. But he's somewhere in here." I offered to go find Gordon for him, as it was obvious that he was worried and concerned that I was alone.

So, leaving the cart behind, we took off together. We toured the huge store aisle by aisle to no avail. As we went up one aisle and down the other, I began to feel sorry for Dr. Caldwell. He only wanted a shovel in the first place. As time passed and we failed to find Gordon, my memory deficits became obvious. I now had no idea where he had gone in the first place, or that I was supposed to be watching a cart, or why I was even there.

Dr. Caldwell, probably sensing my growing confusion, calmly suggested that we could have Gordon paged over the loudspeaker. I looked up at him, and with no uncertain terms, let him know that, that solution was unacceptable. Using the page would indicate that I might be lost and, for once, I certainly wasn't the one who was lost. Gordon was! I wasn't the one that was worried. Dr. Caldwell was. I quickly assured him that I could and would find Gordon and advised him not to worry. I walked the other way, leaving him to find his shovel. I decided to find a quiet place where I could hide out until I could remember where I'd laid my husband.

Sometime later, Gordon found me. His first words were "Why did you leave the area where I left you?" You should have seen the look on his face when I told him that Dr. Caldwell had come and got me. He asked me where Dr. Caldwell was, and I calmly answered, "I don't know". He just stared at me and shook his head.

It wasn't until my family conference later in the week at the hospital, when Dr. Caldwell and Gordon met face-to-face, that I think either really believed the other was ever there.

There were times when even I began to doubt reality. I don't remember to this day, coming home with a bathtub. But my memory book has the story in it, just as I told it to you, and my business checkbook shows we paid $185.00 for one that day. So it did happen.

I have since come a long way on my journey through the mirror of warped perceptions and skewed emotions. Learning to live with a brain injury was not on my planned agenda, and I continually prayed that a cure would miraculously be found. God was obviously busy with someone who needed answers more desperately than I. There was no cure forthcoming. So I adjusted my prayers, merely asking that it not happen to me again. If I was willing to negotiate, so might God. I rested easier thinking that.

This story actually begins two years ago, as I was finishing my formal outpatient therapy. Nothing meant more to me than to be able to drive again, and I was fighting to retrieve my independence in all aspects of my life. I had already fought my way through rehabilitation and I wanted more than anything else, to let them know I was ready to take on the final challenge. My goal was to be an integral part of a functional family, gain my independence on the road and develop a work program that would challenge me and I could take pride in.

My family had been the hardest hit by my injury. You probably should hear it in their own words. It makes the encounters more meaningful. Perhaps, they can tell you many things I can't, or even some things I wouldn't.

They are like driftwood, remnants of another time, left over from the tidal wave that passed through...different shapes, sizes, textures and strengths, all beautiful, yet driftwood, just the same. Each being affected by the storm of injury and trying to understand what is left, the best they can.

First it is necessary that I tell you a little about all of us before the storm. For it is only if you know who we WERE, that you can genuinely feel for who we are.

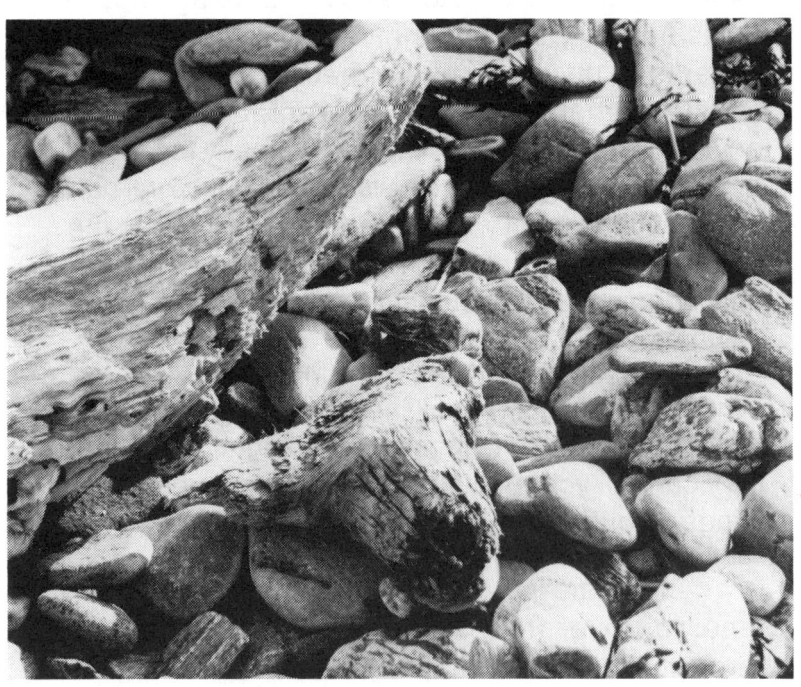

CHAPTER TWO

"Before the Storm"

...From my own perspective...

My family is, and always has been, my life. My husband, Gordon retired from his job as Assistant Superintendent of Schools in the Oxford Hills School District a few years ago. We have made our home in the little southwestern town of South Paris, nestled among the foothills of the White Mountains for the past 21 years. It is a quiet place surrounded by lakes and mountains. We settled here after coming home from an eight-year stint in Rhode Island. We were both native Mainers, from the southern part of the state, but had left for professional advancement.

I met Gordon when we taught together in the same high school where I graduated. He was the head football coach and I coached the cheerleaders.

We were married that summer in 1962 and left for New York University where Gordon earned his Master's Degree. We lived for a year in Piermont, New York in a large house on the Hudson River. I taught at Tappan Zee High School, while Gordon traveled to the city each day for classes.

We left, much to my dismay (as I loved the school), after the school year ended so that Gordon could find a job in educational administration. He became the Principal of a little high school on the coast of Maine. We settled our family in the quaint village of Pemaquid. Well known for its lighthouse and harbors, it was a place that felt good "to come home to". Its natural beauty and total serenity was a stark difference to the urban, fast-paced year we left behind.

I secured a teaching job at Lincoln Academy and Kimberly, our oldest daughter was born, just three weeks before school opened. Those were very treasured, wonderful days. Both Gordon and I loved the sea and spent endless hours just looking outward from the piers of nearby Christmas Cove and from the dock at New Harbor. The smell of the salt air welcomed us home and we rested at night, our stomachs full of newly caught shrimp, scallops, and lobsters.

DOWNEAST TRINITY

*I come to the harbor to hear the sea
and rest and relax at my leisure,
to listen to the downeast tales
that old fishermen tend to treasure.*

*I come in the morning to watch the sea
swallowing sterns of boats, new and old,
with a captain's dream of returning that night
with his catch of the day in the hold.*

*I come to the harbor to feel the sea
to be cooled by the westerly breeze.
I come in the cold with northeasterly storms,
and my jacket pulled tight 'round my knees.*

*I come to the harbor to smell the sea
and wallow in yesterday's bait,
with aroma of fish caught up in the nets
to encounter their inevitable fate.*

*I come at all hours to taste the sea
and all of its gourmet delights,
of lobster served from huge, boiling pots
and clamcakes, Saturday nights.*

*I come to the harbor at dusk and dawn
in winter, springtime and fall.
I come in the heat of the summer crowds,
and I come when there's no one at all.*

*I come to the harbor to share the sea
with the tide, waves and salt in the air.
I come like the starfish, with arms open wide,
clinging to everything there.*

*Just the harbor and me and a wide open sea,
interwoven as part of a whole,
drifting the three of us in an embrace,
in one body, one mind and one soul.*

We stayed in Pemaquid for three years. Gordon and I knew that we would stay there forever, if we didn't seek greater challenges. So our next move took us to the mill town of Livermore Falls, northwest of Pemaquid and inland, very different from the coastal village we left behind.

Gordon became the principal of a much larger high school. I stopped teaching long enough to give birth to Carrie, our youngest. After two years, I began teaching again and we built a beautiful new home on land we cleared ourselves. Gordon oversaw the construction of a new high school and before the dust settled, we got the wanderlust. We planned to go to California, but only got as far as Harmony, a small village in the northwest corner of Rhode Island. Gordon again became the principal of the high school, but Ponaganset was a huge comprehensive high school that had just been completed.

I became quickly involved in coaching and judging the sport of gymnastics. It was an incredibly artistic sport that was new and developing very quickly. Because the rules were in a constant state of change, I was challenged by the never-ending, constant need for knowledge. When there were not enough challenges, I was very adept at making my own. I coached the intramural program, the varsity and junior varsity cheerleaders, girl's cross country, gymnastics, tennis, field hockey, and track and field. I started the "Night of Dance" productions, which was an outgrowth of tremendous student interest.

At the time, most of the physical education programs stressed only team sports, like basketball and softball for girls. I was insistent that my program would be different. I designed programs that were more creative than most. I instituted my own grading program, where students were graded on their participation, rather than their athletic prowess. My students learned things like archery, folk dance, and social dancing, bowling and became recipients of life-long leisure activities. It would be years before this would become common-place in other programs. We started the first co-educational classes in physical education that we had ever seen in the country. Until then, boys were boys, and girls were girls, and God forbid, the twain should ever meet in gym clothes. Folding doors and sliding curtains separated them like enemies. We pulled down the doors and opened up the classes to both, thereby doubling the options of activities offered.

Over the years, I moved into gymnastics judging, instead of coaching. It was more challenging and easier on the body. My judging had spread to other states and I was busy day and night.

Then one night, while at the dinner table discussing family strategies, I casually mentioned to Kimberly that we tended to think like "Downeasterners", more than Rhode Islanders on some issues. She let us know, in no uncertain terms, that she was from Rhode Island and did not regard herself as being from Maine. Gordon and I both looked at each other and for the first time, realized that our next move had to return us home. There is something special about being from Maine, and we both wanted our children to know that specialness and carry on its legacy.

So in 1975, amidst controversy and change, we resettled our family in South Paris, in the heart of an area known as the Oxford Hills. While Gordon was working in the school district, I opened my own crafts business. I watched my children get off the school bus for the first time ever. I had the time to laugh and cry and grow with them as individuals.

I decided I would never teach again. It was too hard saying goodbye over the years to so many students whom I had cherished. I needed to retreat for a while alone. I challenged myself creatively and scheduled time for just me. I was very good at pacing myself and finding my own level of comfort and ease.

Our children were a true blessing. Although they argued and fought like most kids, they were sensitive, intelligent, warm, caring and they "had their heads on straight". We were lucky. Mark graduated from Northeastern in computer math and went on to receive his Masters Degree at the University of Waterloo, in Canada. He has worked for AT&T since he graduated. Today he is a project manager in Malmsbury, England for their UK division. He has bought a home in Bath, England and married Hilary, a beautiful person, inside and out. We now have a British granddaughter and will have another grandchild before you read this.

Kimberly, our oldest daughter, who loves music, theatre, and languages, went to the University of Maine for a career in Engineering. She is now a nuclear engineer at the Kittery Naval Base. She was married during her senior year in College and her husband, Patrick, is an attorney. They have three robust, inquisitive and loving children, Derek, Andrew and Jessica.

Carrie, our youngest daughter, graduated from the University of Maine and is a teacher in a multi-age class (K-2) in the neighboring town of East Sumner. She was married this summer to Henry Raymond, a wonderful man who loves her dearly. She has bought her own home and lives just down the street from us.

Our children have brought us many things to be grateful and thankful for. They have been a source of strength and pride for us. I wish that everybody could be as fortunate.

Over the years, I continued judging gymnastics, getting as far as holding an Elite National Gymnastics Judge's rating and traveling all around the country. The sport is still changing as fast as it was 20 years ago. I love the sport, the excitement, the challenge, the travel, the friends and the gymnasts.

In 1986 when my husband was approaching a time when he was eligible for early retirement from education at the ripe old age of 50, we decided we needed to do something else to help secure our financial position in later life. So I read all of the creative financing plans around and we invested in apartment houses. In order to learn more about real estate, we both became real estate brokers and realtors. I loved learning anything. It didn't matter what it was.

We had been real estate brokers for a company for two years and managing our own units for four years, when my accident happened. My gymnastics schedule was in high gear, and the real estate market was flourishing. No one could have ever predicted the two years that were to follow.

After my car accident, I spent a total of four weeks in an acute care hospital and ten weeks in a rehabilitation hospital. The next year was devoted to home and outpatient therapy and constant supervision. I guess this is where my story started to take shape, when I realized that my road to recovery didn't end with learning to walk and think again. By the time I stopped wandering, could take care of myself, and begin to resume my former life, it was obvious that I still had a long way to go. I saw the return of many of my strengths, my good-naturedness, my organizational abilities in speaking and writing, my love of travel and new things.

But even though I improved so much, my weaknesses became more of a problem. I still got over-stimulated, panicked, made questionable spontaneous decisions (if I made any at all), had trouble pacing myself, and had no endurance. My mind could dream up many things for me to do, but my body couldn't always follow. I still got distracted, and was plagued with impatience.

My brain injury has, also, had a tremendous effect on my family and friends. Up until recently, I was not conscious of how much.

Our family functions differently. We are surviving, but the toll is beginning to show. Maybe it is time to look at things from their perspective.

Since Gordon was the one who had to deal with me on a day-to-day basis, he, obviously, was the hardest hit by my injury. When he offered to give his perspective on my brain injury, I was surprised because he is a very private person and rarely shows his emotion. But living with a wife who has a different personality ,has been a real experience for him. His trek through brain injury recovery has been one full of conciliations, change and constant awareness.

CHAPTER THREE

From Gordon's Perspective

Bev and I had always been equal partners in all aspects of our marriage. Over the years she told me how much she respected me for my honesty, integrity and work ethic. I respected her for her intelligence, decisiveness and common sense. She always did things much differently than I, and maybe that's why we were so happy. When making decisions, I would think things out ahead of time. Bev would decide on the "spur of the moment". I would want our vacations planned well in advance. She would be satisfied with a general time schedule, and living each day as it came. I wanted organization to my daily chores. Bev took what came and did it. I made judgment decisions based on experience and logic. Bev made them on intuitions and feelings. She recognized that I had traits that she lacked, and she had traits that I lacked. Together we made a good team.

We agreed on the most important things in life, like how to make love grow. Whether it was how to *raise our children, or when to fertilize and water the garden, or how to enjoy each other's differences. We cherished the time we had together, and yet, equally enjoyed the time we were apart.*

Bev ended an abbreviated teaching career as a physical education teacher at a high school where I served as principal. She enjoyed all kinds of sports, as well as the arts. I could not have found a better teacher and was proud to have her on my professional staff. It was obvious that she was an inspiring teacher to her students, and they had a special relationship with her. I took great pride in her many accomplishments. Her programs were quality ones, and her sport teams won championships. She could bring order out of chaos, just by her calmness and cool head.

I had obligations to attend meetings, dances, dinners and socials. Bev and I were not just husband and wife, but constant companions.

When she left teaching, she took charge of the house and spent much time with our children. She also spent long hours on the road judging gymnastics and creating stuffed animals for her crafts business.

Upon my retirement from school administration, we went into the real estate business as partners. Being a new endeavor, it was a challenging time for both of us.

When the hospital called me about the accident that resulted in her brain injury, I didn't know *what to expect. I rushed to the hospital emergency room to meet the ambulance. She didn't know my name or where she was. She was admitted right away. It was hard on me mentally and emotionally.*

Even with the passing of time, I still don't know what to expect. I have had much communication with her doctors and therapists. What I have learned is that NO ONE knows what to expect. I have learned to accept that she will never be the person she was before. I am trying to live with the person she has become. At times, it is not easy. There are times when I just want to say, "I can't take it anymore!" But it obviously would not change or achieve anything. I continue to be amazed at Bev's optimism and motivation, and sometimes, that alone uplifts me.

Our marriage relationship is still a 50-50 one, but it's divided much differently. She cannot do many of the things she did before. Some things she can do, she forgets to do. So my effectiveness and sanity rests on trying to remember to remind her to write things down.

She has worked hard to turn her remaining strengths into new challenges. Her creative talents have come forth in her writing. The hours she spends at the word processor is precious time away from our apartment business, which leaves me with more obligations. Limiting her writing is not the answer. She no longer can do or enjoys doing many of the things we did together in the business. She was the one who loved to redecorate all of the apartments, as the tenants relocated. She took great pride in her finished work. Now it is hard to keep her focused on activities she has little interest in. The apartment business is a complex assortment of a multitude of tasks.

What was once a myriad of enjoyment for Bev has now become overpowering. Bev needs to concentrate on one thing at a time, or she gets overwhelmed. She needs to be constantly reminded to pace herself or she goes in twenty different directions at once.

We once worked together for long hours on end, from early morning until late at night with no break. Now she needs short work periods and frequent rest periods. She has little endurance and tires quickly. When she gets tired or bored she needs redirection to get focused or reminders to rest, otherwise she gets impatient, frustrated or angry.

She used to thrive in confusion. She worked best and functioned more efficiently amidst tons of noise and crowds of people. Now she has trouble with the TV set on and someone talking. I must remember to time what I say to her. If she is reading the paper and I talk, she will forget, not only what she was reading, but that she was reading at all. So I weigh the value of what I want to say to her before I start a conversation.

I learned much about brain injury through her rehabilitation process. I learned through reading, the medical professionals, from other survivors and support systems of other families. I learned the most from personal experience and our own interaction with various issues. What I have learned has helped me to improve communication strategies with her, and that has helped us stay calm and work on problems as they occur. We have learned to adjust as Bev has recovered. Both of us needed to change and adapt. It has not been an easy process.

Bev always had an incredible motivation and drive for whatever she attempted to do. She was stubborn and would never give up. Probably that trait was more valuable to her in her recovery than even she realizes. But it has also been a hard trait for me to deal with at home. Her desire to resume activities before she is ready has been a constant source of uneasiness for me. I am afraid for her, because she does not understand fear. Throughout her recovery Bev has always felt that she was invincible and could do anything, just because she wanted to so badly. In the past, she had always been able to do it. Now her abilities fall short of her desire and motivation. She needs to relearn to recognize that. When she walks alone on the street, I fear for her safety.

This is miniscule compared to the fear I felt when she wanted to resume driving. I understood how important it was for both of us, that she drive again. I needed help and relief from the vast amount of chauffeuring required, yet I didn't know what to expect. Somehow I had to come to grips with both our needs.

Bev was the sole financial planner and bookkeeper of our business. It was very difficult not to step in and take over. When your financial future rests on a bookkeeper with a brain injury, you do some very serious contemplating. It was possible for me to take over the finances, but I didn't know the first thing about a computer. Bev had computerized all of the rents, payments, deposits, receipts, checks, billing, tenant records and had done a more than adequate job before her injury. Now she had trouble remembering how to even turn on the monitor.

Bev struggled to keep up, but it was obvious that she no longer understood what she was doing. Our files became lost and she didn't know enough to tell me. It became evident that our business was in jeopardy. She had struggled silently to try to do things that had become far too complex for her to deal with, and I couldn't provide the help she needed.

Since Bev seldom admitted she was unable to do something, or she didn't recognize that she was unable, I was not alerted to how far behind we had fallen, and how much "in the dark" we had been operating.

Bev had not relearned how to reconcile our checkbook and bank statement. I became aware only when our checks finally began to bounce. I felt more secure when Vocational Rehabilitation services provided us with a job coach to help retrain Bev in her computer skills.

When Bev became sick and needed surgery, I wasn't sure that I could go through the worrying anymore. I knew that Bev was strong enough to survive, but I was reaching the end of my ability to deal with the stress. It was a hard time for me. I had to come to grips with my own vulnerability. Bev had physically weathered her injury. She was getting both medical and psychological assistance to help her cope. I was getting nothing. There was little help offered to family members. I felt alone and in dire need of support. It was my job to inform the rest of the family and friends as to what was happening, and many times, I didn't know myself. But Bev continued to make improvements, and I continued to survive.

It is very hard to let go of the past and begin to rebuild your life. It is hard to let go of someone you love and respect, and watch them struggle to begin again on their own. Marriage to a person with a brain injury is a constant "letting go" process, of your own expectations, fears, dreams and future plans, of your tolerances and frustrations, of compromises, adjustments and readjustments. Eventually you come to realize that the person you married is not the personality you're living with. The person you are living with is not the one you fell in love and .built your dreams with.

Oh! I still love Beverley very much and admire what she is doing and how far she has come. It's quite ironic. I admire in her, the very things that frighten me about her. I respect in her, that need for total involvement; the drive to do whatever she wants. Even with a brain injury, she is still able to do incredible things that others, without an injury, only dream about and that has always been an inspiration for me.

I am trying to adjust to what she can do and what she can't, her changed personality and her new desires, her new dreams and her remaining strengths. I am thankful for the professional help that she has received and how far she has come.

I am still, however, often reminded of how far she has to go. It may happen while we are watching television and she is distracted. I may be reminded during a complicated movie when she becomes confused and loses interest, or on a busy street when she darts into traffic without looking. It may be in a group of people or certain sounds when she suddenly panics and bolts out of the room, or it may be just that "look" of a helpless child that lets me know she is lost in the midst of a crowd, and can't escape. It may be the vacant stare I recognize when she doesn't understand, or her eyes as she tries to sort out and make sense of what is happening too fast. These are the times that remind me of how fragile and vulnerable she still is.

Are these characteristics of all persons who sustain brain injury? I don't know. I only know they affect Bev. So until something more effective rolls around, I will just have to take the time necessary to talk slower to her, make sure she is focused on what I am saying, watch her more carefully and continue to love her.

Relationships are meant to change. We grow and are challenged by change. The kind of change we experience may not always be what we planned. But if we make use of the opportunities provided for us, we can do much with the future.

Bev and I will make our own future. We are fortunate to have a good foundation on which to build. Without that, change becomes threatening. I hope I have shown her there is strength in having someone who cares for her and loves her through the good times and the bad. She has taught me that whatever I want for myself is worth fighting for. Maybe that's what makes our friendship, and therefore, our marriage so strong. We've always been fighters and we've always been the best of friends. That's what makes us able to adapt and change to whatever happens to us.

I am looking forward to the person Bev is becoming, rather than trying to remember who she was. I am happier thinking about the future, than the past. Losing that still hurts a little. I am excited to meet the person she will be, when this is behind us. No one knows what the future holds in store. If we did, the last few years would have never happened.

But good things survive and we have so much to be thankful for. We are still alive. We are still enjoying life. We are still in love. Together, we are living each day to its fullest and trying not to dwell on "what was". We use the past to learn from experiences and to be grateful for the chance to begin again. Bev and I will make our own tomorrow. Whatever happens, we have a great start.

FOR MY HUSBAND

*I hold your hand and walk beside you.
We embrace and I am free.
I lose myself in loving you,
And you get lost in loving me.*

*I see your eyes, and I am happy.
We both think now, in terms of we.
I share the thoughts I know will soothe you,
And, in return, you comfort me.*

*Though we've been friends for ever after,
Almost as one throughout the years,
We've built our home with days of laughter,
Strengthening it in times of tears.*

*Weaving it with love and dreams,
Hardening it with work and care.
What we've built, we've built together,
And no one knows the joys we share,*

*From each new day and years that come
While being married to each other.
I could not have found a greater man
Than you, my lifetime friend and lover.*

SECTION TWO

RIDING OUT THE STORM

CHAPTER FOUR

"THE AWAKENINGS"

My first experience with vocational rehabilitation, (more popularly known as V.R.) was at New England Rehabilitation Hospital. During my recovery, I had been assigned to the V.R. counselor there. His name was Ron Spinella. He had worked with me for a short time while I was an inpatient, evaluating my ability and readiness to return to the work force. He met regularly with the Head Injury Team, reviewed my progress as to work readiness and determined what my proper course of action should be.

He was a good listener. It was a full-time task to just weed out the wide variety of jobs I had been doing before my injury. It was even harder to have me try to decide what I wanted to do. I needed to return to nothing (as far as I was concerned) except judging gymnastics, and that was a foregone conclusion on my part, just as soon as they let me out. It was obvious to him that I was nowhere near ready to re-enter the work force. But it was a goal for the future and to work toward. We just needed to decide in what area of work I could be most productive again. Of course, I thought I could do anything and everything.

"I was a person who thought of every human being as a kind of Peter Pan. If you just pointed us toward the stars, turned us 2 degrees toward morning, we could make our own way. The adventure was the journey and the fun was in getting there."

...but in reality, it wasn't that easy.

Most important to my family's financial security, we owned nine apartment buildings, housing 51 units. I was the principal bookkeeper, financial analyst and investor. Gordon had taken over many of my business responsibilities since the accident. Which of these responsibilities I would be able, or want to return to, would be greatly determined by whether I could drive or not.

So I began the process early with Ron, trying to make him understand the importance of my return to driving. He was one of the few people, at the time, who never ruled out driving as a hope for my future. Although he said it was not known if I could succeed, he felt that we should make every effort to try.

That was enough for me. He felt every client should be given the right to fail. I agreed totally.

One day while I was in his office, he called to see if Alpha One, a service organization that retrains disabled drivers, had any experience with severe distractibility. They not only said, "Yes", but also explained that sometimes people, who are distracted in other environmental settings, are not necessarily distracted within the confines of an automobile. My spirits soared as he related that first bit of helpful information regarding my driving potential. Ron was the first to actually explore the possibility of getting me back on the road and giving me hope. At least I had a chance.

Ron never alluded that it was anything more than a chance, but I could live with that much. As I tearfully explained that I needed to be given that hope, for an opportunity to fail if need be, he nodded his head in agreement. But he responded very quickly with the fact that I was no where near ready yet. I needed help with my cognitive deficits.

I would need to work hard on them, even for years if need be. Right now I needed to be patient. I needed to put all my efforts into trying to correct as many problems as I could. He understood my need to try. I knew he felt that I deserved that right to attempt, whatever the odds, as long as it was safe. I had worked hard for that right. But I had no intentions of failing.

He wished me luck and I spent months with the

speech therapist working diligently. When the time came, I was transferred to the neuropsychologist at the hospital. Ron assured me that if I needed him, he would be there to help. I began working with a motivation that no one could stifle.

Dr. David Marks was the new chief neuropsychologist at the hospital. I was assigned to work with him when I had finished all of my other therapies. It had been a year and a half since my discharge from the hospital as an inpatient. I had progressed incredibly. In fact, I had surprised many people with how far I had come during my outpatient therapy.

Dr. Marks was to work with my emotional and coping strategies and try to work on specific deficits that prevented my return to driving. It had been almost two years since I had been behind the wheel.

I told him I could do anything, if he would only find out what was wrong and tell me what to do to correct it. If he would just supply the directions, I would do all the work. I thought that was a pretty simple assignment for him. I'm sure he looked at it differently and much more realistically. But for those with brain injury, getting back to driving takes on a magnified importance, regardless of obstacles faced.

DISTRACTIBILITY

Every now and then,
When I try to bring things back,
My brain goes into reverse gear
And seems to "jump the track".
I want to think of certain things
That I need to achieve,
But my brain does other things
That you would not believe.

Different movements catch my eye,
And stop me in between,
Distracting me to look away
To other things I've seen.
I can't remember where I was,
Or make myself go back,
If my brain forgets itself,
And decides to "jump the track".

They say I should stay focused,
In all the things I do.
It's easier said by someone else
Than trying to follow through.
I set my goals. I gear myself
To concentrate and try.
But then before I know it,
Something else has caught my eye.

So I have just resigned myself,
To take one step at a time.
My brain can go wherever it wants,
And leave the track behind.
I no longer plan to worry
Where my thoughts will go,
And if I get lost wandering,
Hopefully, only I will know.

My first meeting with Dr. Marks was on the day I was to be discharged from speech therapy. He was scheduling me for neuropsychological testing to better ascertain my strengths and weaknesses. He asked a lot of questions. Some I knew the answer to: some I did not. I found it hard to pay attention to anything or anyone for any length of time. He has told me since, how bad my attention skills were on that day, and that he doubted that I could recover enough to ever drive again. But he said nothing to me about my prognosis. I agreed to take all of his tests, provided that if I failed, he would not give up on me. He needed to have faith in me, because I knew I could improve as long as I had help.

The truth was that I didn't like changing therapists. I wasn't sure that I wanted to spend much time with this guy. I didn't know how much he knew, especially as far as I was concerned. Only people who knew me, worked well with me. I didn't trust most people to be able to help me. I answered his questions as carefully as I could, but saw little hope of this man being any help. I knew that I had no choice of therapists and had to make the adjustment. God! I hated change since my accident, especially losing people that I learned to trust.

"Not understanding that change is inevitable as the tide, makes it an ongoing conflict.

Knowing that change is as inevitable as the tide, doesn't make change any easier."

He assigned me to volunteer at the hospital in various jobs and areas. It was a pathway back to the successful work experience. He would assign me to jobs where I had to stay focused in quiet surroundings. Then I would volunteer where I had to stay focused in distracting environments. Dr. Marks scheduled many of my assignments so that they were sequential with my recovery and would challenge me in many different areas where I needed help. All of my work was geared to preparing and allowing me to return to driving.

I filed. I alphabetized. I copied. I learned how to organize and acquired new skills. My jobs advanced over time from simple tasks of filing, to complex areas of word processing programs. Dr. Marks discussed them all with me to carefully assess how I was doing.

I was pleased with how far I had come, by the time I had started working with him. I no longer wandered. I was able to be independent in most things, and my formal therapy was behind me. I had not been able to convince my doctors at the hospital to refer me to Alpha One, but I knew Ron Spinella was waiting for Dr. Mark's approval.

My neuropsychological tests showed that I had severe attention problems, inability to distinquish essential information, judgment problems, severe memory deficits and was much too distractible to be allowed back on the road. It would be a while before the recommendation would even be considered and we had a lot of work to do in the meantime. Dr. Marks assured me that he would keep working with me until

I gave up. I assured him that I would never give up, so victory seemed a sure thing...at least to me. If he could work on finding a way to teach me to scan the environment and yet, stay focused, the door was open to his recommendation. But deep down, I could tell that the door was very close to being locked.

We began by working on problems I found in my gymnastics judging assignments. In returning to judging, I had difficulties remembering some of the things that had been automatic for me before. We developed strategies of making original lists to keep on my clipboard and checking them off as the duties were done. I worked with neon pink scoresheets, because I had learned in therapy to stay focused and relaxed with that color. I used reminders that only I knew about, and placed my chair in odd places to accommodate my visual field deficits. I faced the gymnastic apparatus from different angles to help facilitate visual processing, and to cut down the distractions from the stands. I even wore earplugs during some events to escape from the noise.

No one in the gymnastics field knew the extent of my impairments. Dr. Marks and I worked together on them and made it through the season without any complaints or inquiries. He worked on finding ways to utilize my strengths to make me more functional. I shared my frustration with him of trying to cope with my new self. He helped me understand that my success depended on how I could continue to function in the real world. But like I said before, I was functioning like a different person than before.

*I want to come. She needs to go.
I want to ask. She needs to know.
I want to live. She wants to die.
I want to drive. She hopes to fly.*

Much of our time was spent helping me understand the changes I was living with and how they affected my actual living experience.

We worked in therapy for six months, dealing with daily problems I found in gymnastics. We also worked on the emotional crises that arise after every brain injury, hoping that resolving these would help prepare me for driving.

I purchased attentional software programs for the computer to help stay focused while practicing at home. I bought driving simulation software to get me used to working with distractions. I was assigned to play specific video games every night. I hated them, but my husband diligently saw that I was faithful. Gradually my eye-hand coordination began to improve, and I became better at ignoring the distractions that occurred. Whether it was game familiarity or improvement, I guess we'll never know for sure. But I now firmly believe that some specific games I played had a definite effect on my ability to scan.

I visited all of the arcades and places where they had driving machines. I practiced on them all. Some I did without too many problems. Others, I bombed. But I practiced without exception. Even on evenings when Gordon and I would go to the movies, I would leave him in the ticket line and go to the driving machines. I improved in many of my therapy skills. Dr. Marks was pleased. He had me do verbal skills to help my brain switch gears and I practiced them diligently until I had mastered them all.

Dr. Marks was amazed at my determination. He said he had never worked with anyone who showed that much motivation before. I took it as a compliment. He was becoming successful in helping me and that was what I wanted. We worked well together. He didn't pull any punches and I knew what he said was true. He talked to me about why things happen after brain injury and what changes needed to be made to compensate for things I was no longer able to do.

I listened patiently to what he had to say, knowing he was talking about the changes in me. There were times when the frustration was overwhelming and even though I continued to smile to everyone, I lost faith in the seemingly endless process. I wanted to drive so badly and I felt like getting permission to drive was my only goal. I had to meet special criteria and do certain things before I could get a chance to even try. I was not in control of my life anymore. That was frightening. Dr. Marks had become the umpire, and every day I was constantly stepping up to the plate trying to prove myself worthy.

Brain dysfunction is much like a ball game, but it must be perceived through the eyes of one who is playing it.

PLAYING WITH BRAIN INJURY

I don't remember Willie Mays. I never read Thomas Wolfe either. I want to take my head and go home again.

My body is rounding first base, but my mind is taking the seventh inning stretch. I need to rub my brain with rosin. Sometimes I cannot make it do what I want. I fight it...and it fights right back.

I am always saying to the coach, "Why did I say that? I didn't mean it." He looks at me from a perspective that only I should understand, yet I don't.

I want to steal with the next pitch, so I can be somewhere else, where no one knows my limits. I could be "on deck", or in the "hole", and no one would need to worry. I'd still be safe. But I can make it, if they'd just let me do it on my own.

The rest of the team has sacrificed so that I could walk. I need to give it my best shot, but sometimes, my best shot isn't good enough and my confidence strikes out.

Please coach, I'm calling a "time out". I need to rest. No more double-headers or night games. I need places with no bright lights, no whistles, no noises, no time limits, no scores, no crowds, no stress and no umpires. I don't like games anymore.

There was something very important I needed to remember before the game started, but I have forgotten what it was already. It may have been the batting order. I need to know THAT now, not later after the inning is over.

I try to do things myself, yet when I make an error (and I always seem to), there is no attempt left...and I've been distracted.

I want to plant myself on the base line and watch for signs from the third base coach. But if I should forget what I'm doing, they'll think I'm wandering. There are too many people in the stands watching right now to experiment.

Hundreds of voices from my own team are cheering me on, but if I listen I'll forget the count. I try to stay focused, but something always gets in the way. The voices are still cheering, but I'm not sure what they are cheering for anymore.

The scoreboard says it's two for me and one for you. I can't help but wonder if they're giving me a handicap. I don't want any handicap. I can make it on my own.

I plan to play left field next fall and roll in the leaves of the outfield, losing myself in piles of new-fallen reds, oranges and golds. Breathe in the smell of seasons passed. Some things from long ago, I remember SO vividly.

I earn my uniform of acceptance every day. I relearn the rules and try so hard to win. They *keep telling me to be a good sport and accept my losses graciously.*

I don't need any moment of glory. What I do need is the chance to stand at the plate and determine for myself, when I will swing and when I let things pass.

While the A.L. and the N.L. fight it out to see which league goes down, my AFO brace holds on for dear life, to keep me up. Sometimes, that's all I have.

Just like E.T., I want to go home. Just like Willie Mays, I'd even steal home. Please, Thomas Wolfe, I want to go home again. But I want to go home again on MY terms. I don't need the cheers of the spectators, but I do need the rest of the team to trust me and have faith that I will make it.

I think the "hit and run" is on, or was it the bunt? Does that signal mean I am supposed to run with the pitch or run with the hit? Think! Don't take off without thinking. Maybe I shouldn't run at all. If only I could remember. What if I don't make it?

GO!...Oh No! He missed the ball. Now what do I do? Quick...decide. Make a decision...ANY decision...ANY DECISION!

Oh God! You can have my head. I just want to go home. . . . .

So that is how having a brain injury is very much like that ball game. Survivors are often placated with false promises and reassurances. I was fortunate that my therapists were honest with me. Sometimes, I resented that honesty, but as I recovered I learned to trust them.

I dealt with frustration from dealing with my own deficits, from others who need to change how they dealt with me, and from having to deal with my new self. I also experienced the joy and rewards from knowing that I was becoming more knowledgable and successful in recognizing and handling my own needs. But it would be very untruthful to tell you that recovery isn't frustrating.

After eight months of therapy and work with Dr. Marks, I had gone without driving for two and a half years. I felt that I had improved in every area that we had worked. I wanted an answer. If I was never going to be able to drive again, I needed to make plans to get on with my life. What my future plans would be, depended on my ability to drive. I told Dr. Marks that I needed to find out now. I felt he needed to make a move and make the recommendation for me to be able to try the test. He finally agreed to recommend to Dr. Caldwell that I be allowed to apply for the driving re-entry program.

My next visit was with Ron Spinella. He advised me to contact the State Vocational Rehabilitation Office in Lewiston, Maine, which serviced my home area and apply for services. He gave me the phone number and suggested I make the call myself. I did.

CHAPTER FIVE

TURNING OF THE TIDE

It took a long time to get my first appointment with the State Vocational Rehablitation Services. I thought the time would never come, and that it was an invisible organization that existed only in the minds of other people. My husband became very frustrated over his inability to reach people and the endless amount of phone calls to people who were never "in" and who never returned calls. If he was having this much trouble, I could just imagine what survivors of brain injury who had no support teams to help them, were going through. He complained to the Commissioner and we quickly learned that the squeaky wheel gets the grease first.

When I finally received my date for an appointment, my plan was to apply for funds to assist me in my return to driving with Alpha One.

Once I arrived, I was told that I was probably eligible for total services. I would have to fill out tons of paperwork, and have my doctors fill out even more.

That was fine with me as long as I was eligible. I would be more than happy to do the paperwork. Once I had my appointment, vocational rehabilitation became friendly and supportive to my needs.

My counselor in Lewiston, Pam Williams, was a young, very experienced woman who was extremely knowledgable about procedures and services. Gordon dropped me off at her office, as he had another appointment. I answered all of her questions. The meeting ended abruptly with her asking me, if there was anything else that she should know about my recovery or injury, that I hadn't mentioned.

I told her that I was very prone to panic attacks since my injury. If I heard alarms, sirens, or sudden sounds of someone in distress, I would have an attack. Other than that, I said she need not worry. I could take care of myself. (I think she doubted that, after reading my medical records.) Just as I finished getting the words out of my mouth, there were a series of defeaning crashes directly behind the wall where she sat, with loud constant screaming coming down the wall. A client, with a full leg cast, was falling head over heels down the narrow stairway directly behind her chair. The room suddenly filled with ear-piercing screams.

I don't know what my face looked like, but I saw Pam's. She jumped out of her chair and ran around the desk, put her arms around me so tightly that it was hard to breathe. She said, "We'll walk together out the back way, NOW, GO!". After phoning Gordon from a room in the rear of the offices to pick me up, she walked me around the back of the building and along the side of the parking lot. By that time, the ambulances were pouring in. Pam just kept repeating, "Don't turn around!" She stood with me, hand in hand, on the side of the road until my ride came. We talked about things that had no relevance to the commotion going on behind us. She made very sure that she kept talking and I didn't turn my head to observe. It was a scary and exciting beginning for my vocational rehabilitation--for them and for me. I was to be Pam's first traumatic brain injury client.

The purpose of my second meeting with Pam, was to set up goals for my program. She made sure that Gordon came with me this time. I think Pam felt much more relieved. She asked me what I would like to do for a goal. I answered her very quickly. "I want to write a book." She appeared taken aback. Looking at Gordon for assurance, she turned and said, "No, Bev. We need a realistic goal". I looked over at Gordon for help. "You used to be a real estate broker and teacher. You can't do that again, but you might be able to be a secretary", she continued. I answered her, "I want to write a book". Pam took my hands in hers, turned my head so that I focused on her face, looked me right in the eyes and softly said, "Beverley, if you could write a book, I would eat it."

I lowered my head. Then without interruption, she explained the valuable role of being a secretary as she wrote that on my plan. I had failed to come up with a goal that was realistic for my Individualized Work

Plan. Now it was decided for me. She wrote out my long term goal to become a secretary, stating how VR would assist. I signed the plan confirming my agreement.

The plan agreed to assist me in getting back my driving skills based on Dr. Marks' evaluation and prognosis. We also agreed that VR would provide on-site help with relearning my computer skills. I desperately needed help learning how to operate my computer. I had strong computer skills before my accident. Now I had trouble even turning it on. I knew nothing about the software programs I'd used for years, or the mechanics of operating the hardware. I was assigned a job coach who would work nights with me in my home, getting me reoriented to my computer and rental program. Hopefully I would someday be able to independently return to being the bookkeeper of our business. That was a real goal that needed to be addressed and soon. Our rental business was falling apart financially.

I felt VR was going to be of benefit in getting me back to productive work. But first, I wanted my husband to know in the car going home, that he had just become married to an AUTHOR. I WAS going to write a book. I would prove it to everyone that I was much more capable than they gave me credit for. I would show them I could do anything I set my mind to, and my mind was set. Of course, I had no idea how this was going to happen.

Many people have since asked me how I ever

thought of writing a book in the first place. The idea was originally planted while I was volunteering at the hospital by Donna Levesque, my friend and nurse in the head injury unit.

I had been reprimanded by another therapist earlier for answering the hospital telephone while volunteering. We had dealt with telephone skills on a one-on-one basis for several months in therapy. I thought I had made significant improvement. On my first day of "assigned" volunteering, my task was to clean out a cabinet and not to get distracted from my task. The phone in the room where I was working began to ring. The therapist had stepped out and I hate ringing telephones. So I picked up the receiver and as I was putting it to my ear, I knew I should say, "O.T. East" or "O.T. West", but I wasn't sure which I was in. I made an instant decision to say just, "Hello". I was glad that I had made such a fast decision and solved the problem as well. The phone call was only one therapist looking for another. I offered to take a message and identified who I was. I was proud of how well I had done on the phone.

When I went to my own therapy session that day, my therapist said that she had heard that I answered the phone that morning. I was ecstatic that I had done such a good job and smiled and said, "Yes." I was proud of my job. She let me know that I was not to answer the hospital telephone under any conditions. She said "What would youI have done if it had been the family of a patient? I was traumatized, disillusioned and distraught. After I left the session, I started to cry. I continued to cry for two days. Finally Gordon couldn't deal with me anymore. He led me to the den and turned on my computer and told me to type out my feelings in hopes that it would, somehow, stop the tears. All I could share with him was that no one really understood. No one really trusted me to do things correctly, that it was all hopeless and how tired I was of trying to please everyone. Their placatings were all part of the game. My fingers flew over the keyboard as my thoughts escaped their caged up walls. What appeared on the screen was a three-page expression of feeling that I entitled, "From The Inside Out". I felt better when I finished. It didn't solve any magical problems, but when I looked at the monitor and read, it expressed how I felt. I thought that I had accurately expressed my dilemma, even if it was to an inanimate computer. Gordon helped me print it.

The next day I showed it to Donna. She insisted that I continue writing and putting my story on paper and write a book. I laughed at her. I said, "For God's sake, Donna. You know I have a brain injury. I can't remember what happened ten minutes ago, never mind trying to write a book". She didn't laugh, but the conversation ended. I think it was probably the very first time in my life I had ever admitted that there was something I couldn't do.

When Pam surprised me at my vocational rehabilitation meeting, by asking me what would be a good goal to work toward, my mouth just automatically answered, "Write a book". I believed I could do most other things, and that was the first thing I really believed

I couldn't do.

Deep down though, I knew that my deficits prevented me from ever taking on so big a task. I knew that I needed a lot of help on projects. I was pretty good at taking things apart. Putting them back together was impossible. I couldn't seem to grab the whole concept and visualize it.

People had often underestimated my ability and determination to accomplish things, even before my injury. Why should it be so different now? I never liked to be underestimated. So I felt as if I had to prove everyone wrong. It wasn't the nicest response to take, but sometimes I reacted without thinking of the best solutions.

I seemed to always ride the waves of disbelief and doubt, trying to show people that conquering those waves is 1% ability and 99% motivation and desire. I always believed that percentage.

I had learned in therapy to never let on that I thought I couldn't do something. I would just do it. I didn't know how I could write a book. I would take it one step at a time and figure out each step ahead of time. I WAS going to write a book and tell people what it's like to have a brain injury, what it is REALLY like, from the inside out. Pam, unknowingly, became my motivation.

She had probably dealt with many clients before me who wanted to write books, and believed they could, but who were not at the point in their recovery where that was a possibility. In fact the more I thought about it, very few people without a brain injury ever write books. But I had always been a different animal. I could do anything, because I believed I could. You just had to give me a reason to try. I would prove to everyone that persons with brain injury need to make their own goals and can exceed other's expectations. Anyone who doubted that in the past, helped give me a reason to try. Pam had convinced me she was worthy of my best effort and I fully intended to exert it. I was sure she would be pleased with the result. It would not be just a book, but a manuscript that would mean something to those who read it. Someday she would "eat my book for breakfast", and I would smile as she digested it slowly.

BRING ON THE WORLD

Challenge me with worldly strife,
So my confidence can grow.
I want to build a manuscript
So others understand and know.
When sages revel in the light
That winds its way to me,
I will share the mysteries
Of how I was and came to be.
Bring on the world and challenge me
So I can stand without the crutch.
If enroute, my life improves
We'll all have learned so much.

CHAPTER SIX

GOING BACK TO THE BEGINNING

George Young became my job coach, and I began the tedious job of relearning my computer program for landlords. I had no idea how to use it anymore, or the information that was on it, even though I had recorded almost two years of work on the program. Since George has never seen the program before, we were like two beginners trying to solve a complicated program. It had been used by me before, had all of my past rental information stored on it, and had just been left in the middle of operations because of my accident.

It felt like I was returning from a vacation and trying to reactivate my operational systems, yet I couldn't remember how. I didn't understand the concept of the software. I didn't recognize any of the information that I had recorded in the past. Worse, I had no idea how to find out. Since George was new to my rental business, he didn't either. He took the tutorial for the rental program home and did his homework. When he returned, we experimented with the beginnings of the program. I remembered only two things, which must have been things that I overlearned because of their importance. One of them was that you always needed to return to the menu before exiting. The other was that I could not use the control/alternate/delete function to clear the screen, as you could with most programs. Why this information stuck in my head in really unknown, except maybe as I said, it was of such importance to me before. After logging about twenty hours of work on the program together, I found myself in the wrong application area. George suggested I push the control/alternate/delete and start over. Bells went off in my brain and triggered an alert. "NO!", I told him quickly. "You can't do that." He assured me that it was okay. I told him I didn't know why, but we couldn't do that. He reached over my shoulder and pushed the three keys simultaneously.

We lost everything. The screen, the information, the input and the whole program was deleted from the disk. I was not as surprised as George. Although I didn't remember what would happen, I knew we would be in trouble. While it took me a long time to believe that all the time, work and energy had been lost, it was probably for the better. Not only had it erased all the files, but we had to reinstall the original program on the computer again. I lost all of my old files and information that really meant nothing to me anyway. George and I started from scratch, recording again all of the transactions from the beginning of the year. Repetition was such a good strategy for me, so we learned together.

George was the kind of guy who would do anything for you. He was good-natured, good-hearted, and a happy person. He never came to the house without a smile and a happy disposition, even though he might have had a hard day. I appreciated that trait and it helped me to keep up my motivation for a very boring activity, but one that I knew was essential for my job independence. He turned the tedious and complicated job into a project that I could handle. At least I could process a part of it, and feel like I was slowly becoming of some value.

We began by writing everything down in list form that I had to do. All of the operational aspects of the computer were listed in order, so that I could follow them and check them off as I did it. The list included which keys to press and the order in which to press them. By going back to the beginning, I could feel as if I could do it myself, even though I couldn't yet. I had retained all of my typing ability. My right hand was still not back to normal as far as small motor functioning and finger speed, but it was fast enough to keep up with my slower brain processing. I made out fine as long as I took things slowly and stopped before I went into overload.

George learned quickly to recognize those times when I suddenly stopped functioning, or nights when trying to function was not going to produce any results. He quickly adjusted his schedule, and we tried to make good use of the quality time we had.

Even though we started again with my rental program, we still met many obstacles with it during the next few months. But we repeated, reworked and reread the manuals. George worked with me, and together we began to make progress on my bookkeeping. We worked four to six hours a week on specific tasks. Rent payments, receipts, checkbook items, journal entries, and tenant and unit information became weekly things we handled. I did them with George's help, but at least I did them. My job was to keep all of the receipts and records in one place until he arrived. I did THAT pretty well.

By the end of the year, I was able to perform many of the aspects of the bookkeeping jobs. I still needed help on the choices within the menu, and sorting out complicated decisions. I had trouble with divided attention. I was unable to take my eyes away from the screen to do another task, and then return my attention to the monitor and continue. So George did one task, while I did the other.

I became aware of how much George helped me by trying to work alone without him. I was unable to work by myself without getting totally lost. When it came time for income tax reporting, for instance, I found I had major problems. I had no idea what figures went where, and into what categories the totals went. For instance, should money spent to repair glass be considered maintenance, or should it be considered repairs?. There were almost 50 categories in my program and only three for I.R.S.. I had major problems in making any decisions. I totally gave up and just made random decisions. I kept no list of where I put things, so when my books went to the accountant, I had no idea where anything was. I was helpless and I'm sure he thought I was hopeless. I had been totally honest and had spent endless hours keeping meticulous records, but if I ever got audited, because of my memory deficits, I would have to admit I had no idea where anything was. I confided in George that I was concerned, and he understood. It was useless to spend the time that we were, keeping accurate books, if I didn't know what to do with the information once it was accumulated. We had worked over 14 months relearning a program that was not working for me. At this rate I would never be independent.

Our time had been valuable and necessary for my relearning, as I had regained many of my computer skills in the process. I had become familiar once again with my bookkeeping and my business. I had learned to use the software methodically and understood the hardware.

George began to work with me on condensing categories, thereby making the decisions easier for me to deal with. So I started again to learn new categories, new accounts, and the process began all over again. I was good at breaking things into segments in order to better understand them. Time would tell if it worked.

SEGMENTS OF RECOVERY

a time for wondering where you've been..
a time for working on how it'll end..
of missing links and broken chains..
of so many losses and so few gains..
a time for almost, but not quite..
a time to struggle day and night..
a place of many childlike pretenses..
a place to hide and soothe the senses..
a time to think, but not to know..
a time to wander, but not to go..
one of encores and repeat performances..
a time for being not in accordances..
a second to wish and an hour to cry..
a time to laugh and then wonder why..
a helping hand to recoup the past..
a time to pray that it won't last..
a time to try and try and then..
a time to try and try again..
a time to follow, but not to lead..
fighting the struggle to hear and read..
a time to relearn what I'm about..
finding my best time is "time out"..
a time I never thought I'd see..
a time to build another "me"..

CHAPTER SEVEN

TAKING THE WHEEL

While I worked with my job coach, Dr. Marks continued to work with me on my cognitive problems to return to driving. At the same time I was struggling to relearn my computer program, the day arrived for my driving evaluation.

I became nervous that it was going to be an exercise in futility. Maybe everyone had been right. Did they know that I was unable to handle driving and weren't telling me? Maybe I had overestimated my ability and just didn't realize it. I had been known for doing that over the past two years. I wasn't sure what I would do if I failed, because I never let myself consider that possibility, at least out loud.

I packed all my fears, along with my prayers, in my pockets and started out. The day was finally here. Gordon drove me to the agency on that day for testing, and waited as I anxiously walked into their office for my evaluation.

The person asked me for a history of my problems. They had not received any of my records from the hospital, doctors, or vocational rehabilitation. I had the privilege of supplying my own version of my deficits. I gave them an overview, with a watered-down version of what problems I had had. I may have suffered a brain injury, but I was never stupid. I didn't feel at all guilty about not telling them everything I had trouble with. We would have been there all day and I didn't know for sure which deficits, if any, were relevant to my driving. There was no need to worry about what might not even happen.

She gave me some perceptual tests that I thought I did well on. Then she took me on the road for a driving test. We drove in moderate traffic conditions in the city and on roads in the surrounding rural areas. We practiced turns in an empty parking lot. I listened to everything she said as carefully as I dared, without losing focus on the road. I was very careful to turn my head to the right to compensate for my visual field deficits diagnosed earlier by my doctors. I felt I did really well considering. I made a right hand turn and hit the sidewalk, but she said nothing.

One of my worries was that, even should I pass, I would be restricted to daytime driving, or limited to driving only so many miles from home, which would not be of any help to me in returning to gymnastics or my volunteer work at the hospital. When we finished the actual driving part of the examination, we returned to the center and talked. She told me that I should practice for 5 hours with a licensed driver. That was standard procedure for all. The Department of Motor Vehicles would be scheduling me for a road test and would contact me with a date. She also said that the agency would be recommending no limitations on my license.

I wanted to grab her and hug her, but I just thanked her politely. I felt a sudden surge of pride for having pushed myself further than others thought I could or should. I felt a pride for daring to do things and not just dreaming about them. I felt a pride for all the times I stayed inspired and motivated, and didn't let the work get me down. It was a total pride for refusing to take "No" for an answer and never giving up.

When I returned to the hospital with positive results, I could see the fear and apprehension in everyone's eyes. Even though they had been encouraging me and keeping my spirits up through the long months, I knew deep inside that most felt I would never drive again. But that was okay, I understood their concern. They cared.

I waited for three weeks for the state to notify me of a date for testing. After not hearing from them, I called the Medical Review Board directly to get an answer. They said I had been cleared by their board the week before and NO road test would be necessary.

I laid down the phone, turned to Gordon and

smiled. He knew. He was not as happy as I was, but he tried not to let me see it. He knew that there would be no holding me back. Dr. Marks had been successful and I had worked very hard, too. Now the fruits of our efforts would pay off.

The very next morning, I drove the 50 miles to the hospital alone. Gordon nervously kissed my cheek and watched me drive out of the driveway. I knew he was holding his breath, but I was sure I could do it on my own. I was determined to begin immediately.
That was exactly what everyone was so worried about.

Gordon lived with me every day and saw the changes in me and helped me find solutions. He understood that I was different than before my injury. He supported me in whatever I dreamed up to do and tried to change with me.

Kimberly, my oldest daughter, saw my injury in a different perspective. She saw me less often and wanted her mother back. While driving was my priority, it was not so in her perspective. In fact, it was the least of her concerns.

CHAPTER EIGHT

FROM KIMBERLY'S PERSPECTIVE:

I'm Bev's oldest daughter and I have a different perspective than the rest of the family about my Mom's injury and and recovery.

I guess everyone looks up to their Mom. I know I did. She was amazing. She could answer a million questions at once and help me deal with success and loss (whether it was accepting a boy's class ring or the death of our dog). She would always understand and help me cope when I needed her.

I remember when I first heard of Mom's accident. I was eight months pregnant with my third child. I was concerned that no one would tell me the truth about Mom's injuries. I felt that Dad and the rest of the family were watering everything down. Even when I went to visit Mom, she insisted she was fine. It wasn't true. She couldn't hold an orange or remember my husband's first name.

When Mom entered the rehabilitation hospital, I was hurt. A regular hospital fixes things and then discharges you. What was a rehabilitation hospital supposed to do? "Retrain", they said. I didn't want my Mom retrained, especially by strangers! They didn't know my Mom before. How could they teach my Mom how to act? They didn't know how she acted before. I wanted to stay there until she got well, but I couldn't. I had to work until my maternity leave, and the two hour trips to the hospital were not doctor-recommended. Even with pregnancy, I had two small boys who were a loving handful. I felt guilty that I couldn't be there for my Mom.

Once Jessica was born, I found out more and more about Mom's injury. Dad was very protective of Mom and tried to explain her limitations and need for quiet time. As I listened, I thought, "Quiet time? What quiet time? The only quiet time I have is between the 1 A.M. 'Can I have a drink of water?' and the 3 A.M. feeding".

My mom always had the job to understand and I had to cope. After Mom's injury, it became my job to understand and HER job to cope. The trouble was that I didn't understand. "Let her out of that chair! Mom, where are you?" I wanted my real mom back, yet I didn't even know where she had gone.

The feeling I had leaving her at rehab was similar to the guilt felt by a working parent when leaving a child at daycare. But at daycare, I knew the providers I received daily progress reports.

They all knew my name. My children were happy at daycare, but I felt my mom was not happy.

During the past four years, Dad has reminded me to try to keep things simple. "Simple? How can my family fit into her life now?" I work full-time as a nuclear engineer, while my husband, Patrick, works different and long hours as an attorney. I co-chair our PTA and work in the school computer lab. Patrick coaches in the recreational league and is on the town's Board of Appeals. We now have three small children that keep us on the go. Derek and Andrew both play soccer, basketball, baseball, and hockey, as well as academic after school activities. Jessica takes dance lessons and plays soccer. We cart all three children to lessons ranging from ice skating to swimming, depending on the season. We are planning house renovations and on any given day at 5 P.M., our house makes the New York Subway System seem quiet.

I have always said that when my husband gets sick, it's like having four children, but in a way I was kidding. Now I have 5. There are times when I feel like my Mom and I have reversed roles. I filter or simplify things for my children and now I must watch what I say to Mom.

My children have no problem with their "new Gram". They are too young to really remember the old Gram. They accept that she needs her memory book, because they love to color and write things down, too. When she couldn't drive, neither could they. They are good about taking her hand when crossing streets, because they know she forgets sometimes to look for cars like they do. They understand that. They also understand that she is prone to forget other things, and so they are quick to remind her, two or three times, what they want for their birthdays and Christmas. We make and send lists of scheduled soccer games and other events.

What the kids don't understand is why we don't visit as much. They don't understand why their 83 year old great-grandmother can answer lots of questions quickly and babysits a lot, but Grammy Bryant doesn't. They don't understand why Grammy Bryant suddenly disappears at birthday parties, cries at Thanksgiving, and takes naps at Christmas.

It's hard for me to deal with, too. Mom seems so normal at times. I'll start to believe that she's back. Then suddenly with a bit of confusion, a decision or two, or noise, she turns into a child. I can't leave the kids alone with Mom for any length of time. Children, as we all know, are walking complications, questions, dares and demands.

Being an engineer, making decisions is my life. That's what I do. I gather facts, use logic and make decisions. I can't imagine losing that ability. I've known people who are indecisive. Neither Mom nor I could tolerate them very well. I always knew I inherited my decision-making skills from my Mom. I was always taught that avoiding decisions was a cop-out. I guess I can't accept my own Mom, of all people, copping out.

Mom and I used to drive weekly to music lessons and we would sing, debate current events and coordinate upcoming schedules. I miss her organized chaos. I loved her "juggling" skills. My Dad contemplated, wrote lists, and completed doing everything in that order. He always has been steady, prompt and very reliable. My Mom would brainstorm, write down gobs of good ideas on a napkin, lose the napkin, but knew what she had to do and did it in her own way. Mom was the one who was unpredictable. Now she really is.

I love my Mom, even what is left. The person I lost was a maverick, yet she was my stability. She was my bouncing board, my friend, and my vent. I need a vent path at times. Just an incoherent phone call placed randomly, just to say, "Mom, Is this how you survived parenthood?"

The children like to talk to her on the telephone. Yet when I talk with her, something in her voice seems to fade away. To me, she appears to lose interest. I never learned to stay focused with her on one subject at a time. I constantly jump from one subject to another without thinking. I forget she is unable to switch topics and follow me anymore.

If she doesn't write things down, she will probably forget the entire phone call. I pay bills to our phone company and sometimes, for no reason. Who am I talking to? I know my Mom is aware of it and tries to pay attention. It hurts her just as much as it hurts me, if not more.

There are times when I just need a little advice and someone to understand. Mom and I have always communicated well. It's socially acceptable for a married woman to vent her frustrations to her mother. When I had to stop calling Mom and stop bouncing things off her, I lost my best friend.

No one understands my loss. My mom's photo looks the same. She is no longer in the hospital. She still smiles. She didn't die. In fact, most people think she's back to normal at first glance. But to me, a very valuable part of her is gone, and no one but a few, really know. I guess that is the hardest part of all. It is hard to grieve a loss that others cannot see, share or feel.

I've gone through denial, anger, pity and I guess I'm working on acceptance. I can't appeal the decision or diagnosis of a brain injury. I can't go back again and undo what's been done. Anyway you figure it, she'll never be the same to me.

I can scream, cry, and look for reasons, but it won't change the past or present. We can only live today, learn from yesterday and prepare for tomorrow. I'll never forget my "old" Mom. When I recognize her for a few calm minutes, it is comforting to feel her presence.

I've never minced words with my family. When

my Mom would take me shopping, I was the only sibling who would say that the blouse she was about to buy looked like Aunt Daisy's kitchen curtains. My mother dreaded back-to-school shopping with me. Sometimes what I say, hurts, but my family knows that I will tell it to them straight.

This situation is hard though, because we are talking about my mother's brain. It is something she can't exchange for a new one. Over the past four years, I am slowly accepting that it may never be the same for me.

I wish I had appreciated her more. I'll continue to search for the "old bird" I loved so much, while my "new" Mom searches for her wings.

SECTION THREE

AT THE HELM

CHAPTER NINE

RUNNING WITH THE TIDES

As I left my home on my first day of driving, it took me only about 15 minutes to realize that something was wrong. I found that my car would move to the left, as though I had an under-inflated tire on the left side, or the road was tilted to the left. I realized quickly, that the road was level and my tire pressure was fine. It was more difficult for me to see and process things to my right. I tended not to look in that direction, and suddenly things would pop into my peripheral vision that I had not seen coming.

When I stopped at lights and stop signs, I stopped my car far beyond the center line. Several times when stopping at intersections, before turning left, I found myself in the oncoming lane, rather than on the right. Luckily no cars were coming. I recognized the problem AFTER I had done it, but was not aware of it when the problem occurred, so I took no action to prevent it.

When I was about ten miles from home, heading south that morning, I saw an approaching school bus. Realizing immediately that it represented a safety hazard, I began to concentrate on it. I thought to myself that there were apt to be young children running out in the road, and I should be careful to watch out for them. I saw the red lights flashing from the bus and recognized that they meant for me to stop. I slowed down, as the car ahead of me came to a stop.

While I sat looking at the car in front of me, I felt a sick feeling deep in my stomach. I realized I had stopped my car only because the car ahead of me had stopped. I suddenly knew that if I had not been following that car, there was no doubt in my mind that I would have continued on. My brain deciphered that I needed to pay special attention. Once I had recognized that situation, I was unconsciously "done" with it. I didn't understand that I needed to do something else...like react. I never would have actually put my foot on the brake to stop the car. I traveled very slowly on purpose, watching for more schoolbusses, all the rest of the way to the hospital.

My next hint of trouble came as I approached the toll booth exiting Interstate 95 at Exit 7. There was a traffic jam as cars from both North and South exit ramps tried to merge quickly into a few lanes. I couldn't decide which lane to move into. While my brain pondered, my car came to a halt in the middle of six or seven lanes of traffic. I just sat there, my eyes fixed ahead to the confusion beyond. It took three or four minutes probably (which seemed like an hour) to start moving again amidst the cars weaving around me. I felt totally incapable of joining this mass confusion, but knew, also, that I needed to get by.

As I approached the toll booth, I tried to sort out whether to first, take out my toll pass, open my window or take the ticket. My car weaved back and forth, jerked forward as I fumbled between tasks trying to make a decision. It was a horrible experience. Once I had gone through, I frantically threw my pass on the floor. I then tried close my window, accelerate and get into another lane.

Tomorrow, I quickly decided I would drive the back way into the city. I would not take the turnpike again until I could get my act together. Trying to deal with one thing at a time was hard enough. Forget this problem of trying to do six things at once.

That day I met with Dr. Marks. He patiently listened to my morning experiences. I knew he was not as worried about my actual driving ability as much as my ability to handle the incidental parts of driving. But he didn't make any judgments and said we must work on breaking these problems down, if we were going to have any success in solving them.

I practiced saying "flashing red lights" out loud, as I visualized seeing flashing red lights on a school bus, and picked up my right foot and moved it to the left. I did that sequence 80-100 times a day. I never got sick of doing it because I knew it would help me drive more safely. I practiced diligently all by myself, day after day, night after night. I knew that if I was unsuccessful at correcting things, I would lose the right to drive. I had no intentions of hurting anyone else in the process of my relearning. That was motivation enough for me. I had no more problems with schoolbus1es.

      Together, Dr. Marks and I came up with a list of the order of things that I would do, when approaching toll booths. First, I would stay in the lane I was originally in. By not changing lanes, no matter how many cars were ahead of me, it would eliminate one decision. He reminded me that I was never in a hurry so it would help me to wait in a line, by giving me extra time to go over my list. The second thing was to stop the car at the toll gate first. THEN I was to get the pass and roll down the window. Once I got the pass back, I was to put it away, then roll up my window. After that I could drive away slowly, staying in the same lane. I needed to make sure not to make any obscene gestures to those people honking behind me. I had to concentrate on one thing at a time. If people behind me got excited, that would have to be their problem.

HELPERS
Sometimes, I bite my lip
And silently squeeze my fists,
That my life should be controlled
By memory books and lists.
But I laugh and lighten up

*Because in the end, I know,
Without those little strategies,
I would not be apt to go.*

    I affixed the list to my dashboard, so that it was in front of my eyes every day and I followed it without exception. If I didn't succeed it would not be because I didn't try. I was determined to drive. We labored over how I would correct each problem I encountered, and we would devise creative strategies to work them out. Some worked and some didn't.

    I found that once stopped at red lights at intersections, I did not remember to go automatically when the light turned green. Cars behind me would often honk their horns and that would stimulate me to realize that I needed to step on the gas. One of the strategies I devised, whenever I thought of it, was to avoid being the first car in line at the intersection. I felt maybe it was the distractions within the intersection that made me forget, so I always tried to be the second car in line. Then I didn't have to react to the light, when it suddenly turned green. I tended to follow the first car in line, when it started up again. This strategy worked well until about a month or so later. I suddenly found myself about eight miles south of where I had been headed. I said to myself, "What on earth am I doing in this neck of the woods?" Then I realized I was still following the car ahead of me...(oops-end of strategy)....Once I learned a strategy though, it was more difficult to unlearn it.

One day while I was driving, it suddenly started to rain very hard. I couldn't see through the windshield. I knew I needed to see better, so I rolled down my side window. While lifting myself up, I put my whole head out of the window to try to see. As the rain hit my face and my wet hair blew in my eyes, I thought to myself, "There must be a better way to do this. I don't think other people hold their heads out of the window to see when it's raining". It was a time before I figured out about windshield wipers. Then finding them, to turn them on, became an even greater task. But I made it home and Dr. Marks and I worked in therapy on what had happened. After many strategies that didn't work, we discovered a product that when put on the windshield in advance, allowed the water to run off and using the wipers were not necessary. I was to make sure that it was always on my windshield.

One of the exciting things that happened immediately was that once it was on my windshield, the first time it rained, I was able to remember to turn on my wipers. I think what happened, is that this covering made the rain hitting the windshield accummulate in droplets. They stayed in droplet form for a few seconds as they floated across the glass. The sustained cue (of seeing the drops of water) lasted long enough to make a connection in my brain and I had time to figure out what I had to do. I now make sure that my windshield is always protected.

My "Waterloo" almost came when I ran into a

deficit that we found impossible to cure. Dr. Marks said it was related to the same initiation deficit that I had with the wipers. I always remembered to turn on the headlights of the car if it was dark outside when I got into it. But if it became dark while I was already driving, I was unable to remember to turn on the lights. Several times I completed journeys in complete darkness, unaware that I needed only to reach out and turn on the lights. We worked on strategies in therapy to help me try to remember to turn them on. We used colors, audio tapes, songs, alarm clocks, adaptive watches, signs...and nothing worked. I tried to think of creative things that I could use to remind myself or cue myself, but we tried everything and nothing worked.

One day while returning from a conference in New Hampshire, I stopped at my daughter's home about 80 miles south of mine. I called Gordon to tell him that I was on schedule. It was about 6:15 P.M.. His first words were "Please go out and turn on the car headlights right now." I told him that I'd be there for 15-20 minutes and would do it when I left. So that he would rest easier, I said loudly so that he could hear, "Kim, will you go out with me when I leave and make sure I put on my headlights?". Kim answered loudly back, reassuring him she would. I hung up the phone, as Kim took the children upstairs for their baths.

I looked at my watch, concluded that if I left right then, I could be home by the time it got dark and I wouldn't even need my headlights. Yes, that would be a great idea. I left without saying goodbye to my daughter, or kissing my grandchildren, or saying a word to anyone. I started my car and headed North. When I reached Poland, a town about 16 miles south of my home, it was totally dark. I spent the next 16 miles thinking how careful I must be, because I couldn't see. While my mind pondered my predicament, there was NEVER a thought that said, "Reach out your hand and put on the headlights." ...and I never did.

The first time that I considered that had been a possibility was when I walked into my home, an hour later. Gordon said to me, "Hi Hon, Did you turn your lights on okay?" I suddenly realized that that was why I hadn't been able to see well. I mumbled something undistinguishable and kept going. I hadn't recognized the right problem, even though I knew I couldn't see. Therefore, I couldn't determine the right solution. I came to the conclusion that Dr. Marks and I had better get to work fast on the "light" problem, or I would not be on the road for long...initiation or no initiation.

It was hard to talk to anyone about this inability of mine to act when I needed to. Not only was it humiliating in retrospect, but I always feared that there would be no alternative, but to give up my right to drive. I had come too far and worked too hard, and harbored no intentions of allowing that to happen.

The next morning Dr. Marks decided very

quickly that we needed to find another solution beyond strategies. He told me the only way he knew to prevent this danger from continuing to happen was to have my car lights wired permanently to the starter. Then every time I turned on the car engine, the headlights would come on. That way they would automatically be on when it became dark. He spent all morning calling Toyota factories and lighting companies to inquire about the possibilities and their suggestions.

Vocational rehabilitation agreed to cover the cost of having my car permanently adapted to my specific needs. A local company that does work for challenged people who need adapted automobiles, rewired my car's lighting system the next week. End of problem.

I discovered other problems, and we worked equally hard on those. There were several places near the hospital where there would be five or six blocks with a stop sign at the end of each one. Then suddenly, the next block would have a red light instead of a stop sign. I would continually go through the red light. My brain would stay focused on the stop sign and didn't switch gears and look for the light. It took over two months of constantly trying to remember that particular light and using strategies, before I was able to remember to stop at it.

After I had been driving a couple of months, I was in a long line of traffic on a two-lane road. Having a long, open space ahead, with enough room to pass the three cars in front of me, I signaled. Pulling into the left lane, I stepped down on the accelerator. I was aware that I needed to be careful in this situation. As I was passing the first car, I noticed that the car in front of it had its left hand blinker on and it was slowing down. I also noticed a side road to the left, exiting ahead. I said to myself proudly "AHA! This guy doesn't know that he can't make a left hand turn from the right hand lane." I never, for a moment, realized that I was in the wrong lane and he was going to turn left. He turned sharply, as I steered wildly to avoid a collision. I never put my foot on the brake. As I drove my car beside his, we took the left hand turn together on the side road, my car turning at a much faster rate. By the time I realized what had happened, my car was stopped on the side road in the wrong lane again. The other car had disappeared far ahead. I just sat and tried to figure things out. Sometimes I just needed time to think and analyze what I did wrong. This time, I thanked God that I even reacted, especially in such a quick manner. I also thanked him for the fact that no cars were coming in that lane on the side road.

The next day Dr. Marks set up strategies for me to repeat, memorize if possible, write down and follow, so that this type of situation would not reoccur. I was only to EVER pass one car at a time from then on. If there was more than one car, then I would not attempt to pass. I repeated for days, "Pass one car only. Pass one car only. Pass one car only". I also put a large printed note on my windshield that read, of course, "PASS ONE CAR ONLY", so I would not be tempted to forget again. I didn't forget.

I never had any problems putting my turn signals on, or knowing how to start, shift or steer the car. I knew all that. In fact, I knew how to do everything I didn't do. It was just that when the time came, I didn't do it.

In the months that followed, I was the happiest person alive. We worked each week on perfecting my driving strategies. Gradually over the six months of driving and constant therapy, I worked hard to erase many of my deficits that put me, and others who got in my way, in danger of injury. It was not easy and some who got in my way were not always so lucky.

EULOGY FOR A CAT

One afternoon I was on my way home. It was a peaceful day and I was driving slowly North on a long, open stretch of road on Route 26.

Listening to my music softly in the background, I saw movement ahead on the side of an open field. My eyes scanned and settled quickly on this beautiful, large cat that was moving toward the sandy shoulder at the side of the road.

I silently marveled at my new-found ability to scan the environment and how far we had come in dealing with my driving deficits. It was really remarkable.

I wondered who this cat belonged to, so far away from houses. Someone obviously loved it. It appeared to be well-fed and well-cared for. As the cat continued to walk toward the road, and my car moved closer, we seemed to be in tune with each other; each of us moving in our own separate way on our journey homeward.

I felt uneasy that this cat was venturing so near the road. It was lucky that I was driving very slowly. Someone else might have been passing and driving at the speed limit, or even faster, through this stretch and not see the cat, like I had. Or even I might have been hurrying home, like on most days, instead of taking my time to enjoy the scenery.

As the cat walked out directly in front of my car, I said to myself, "Wow, This cat had really better be careful. It must be deaf. Someone might"........CLLLUUUUNNNNNNKKKKKKKKKK!

I was about a half mile down the road, before I put my foot on the brake. The cat was far behind me, and much time had passed before I knew enough to stop my car. It was much too late for the cat.

In therapy the following day, Dr. Marks asked me how my driving was going. I broke down in tears, reluctantly reliving the saga of the cat. I was concerned about how I failed to recognize one, simple necessary action...to step on the brake. I understood what had happened, but I was helpless to find a solution.

He let me cry. He's good like that. He let me have my time to straighten myself out. As I tried to regain my composure, I tearfully asked him, "What would have happened if it had been a child?" He knew he didn't need to answer. It wasn't really a question. He knew what I was sure of. I would have done the same thing.

As I sobbed for what might have happened, and grieved for a dead cat, Dr. Marks looked over at me and said, "Do you think you are having second thoughts about your ability to drive safely?" My mouth blurted, "NO" hardly before he had finished his question. "No", I stated again, as if he hadn't heard me the first time. "No, No, NO!", I added. I wanted to leave no doubts that I was driving and that was final. I had come too far and worked too hard to go down gracefully with honor. They would have to shoot this "Titanic" out of the water, because I was staying afloat, no matter how hard I had to struggle. I was not giving up.[1] He would just have to find a way to make me put my foot on the brake. PERIOD! No more discussion. But first he allowed me the time to cry again, not just for the cat, but for me. And I did, for a long, long time.

---

[1] I have since successfully passed a road test with the Department of Motor Vehicles and made sure I have corrected these deficits.

CHAPTER TEN

THE LAST HURRAH

It was near the end of April, and I was in the middle of the hardest part of my gymnastics season. I was scheduled to judge at the State Championship Meet in a nearby city. I now knew that I needed to use several strategies to do my job of judging.

So I left an hour early, drove along for quiet time, and arrived at the arena in time to be able to study before the meet began. I parked outside and sat in the car, so that I could be alone. Suddenly the Meet Director came running out to my car window and asked if I would go to the florist shop and get some flowers. One of the judges was supposedly retiring, and this was to be her last meet. I said, "Sure, no problem". (Famous last words)

As it was only 8:45 A.M. on Sunday morning, the florist shop was not open, so I made a decision to try to get back into the heart of the city to find another florist shop before the meet started at 10.

    I was driving up a city street, looking for the shop on either side, when I noticed a police car approaching me on MY side of the road. I pulled my car as close to the right curb as I could. As I attempted to pass his car, he opened his door. I slammed on my brakes to keep from running into him as he stepped out. He approached my window, which was open, and started yelling in a loud voice.

    Between his face and mine, less than 24" apart, was my middle finger extended upward. I was mortified. It was not something that I planned to do or had any control over. When I realized what I had done, I didn't even attempt to take it down. I just mumbled repeatedly, "stupid, stupid, stupid." The policeman thought I was calling him stupid, and got even more upset.

    He asked me if I was aware that the road I was on was a one-way street. Once he said that, I remembered that it was and I answered, "Yes". He just looked at me in disbelief. As I broke down in tears, I noticed a brain injury survivor card tucked into my visor and handed it to him. I couldn't stop crying or explain anything.

    He didn't give me a ticket. He told me to turn my car around and GET IT OUT OF THERE. Then he returned to his car and drove off and left me. It took me a while to figure out how to do that, as cars were lined up for a long way up ahead of me, coming in the other direction.

I did get the flowers, but I stopped at a grocery store and bought them on my way back to the gym. By the time I arrived, the competitors were lined up on the floor and the national anthem was playing. The director of the meet was in a state of panic, more over my absence than the flowers.

I learned that sometimes, planning ahead isn't always enough, and changing plans isn't always the best choice. Little did I know then, that that day would be MY last gymnastics meet, too.

I was so humiliated by what had happened that I didn't tell Gordon for a very long time afterward. I did tell Dr. Marks what happened at my next visit and we again worked on ways to prevent it from happening again.

I, also, made a promise to myself that I would see to it that possession of the "alert" cards for persons who had sustained a brain injury were encouraged.

BLUE JELLYFISH

*I've seen large, red jellyfish
And even, some that's white.
I've never seen a blue one
Though I've been warned by some I might.*

*I have interrupted jellyfish
So I have felt their stings.
They look so very innocent,
But they're sleezy, slimey things.*

*My brain is like a jellyfish,
soft and jiggling, if I shake it.
Swimming in my boney skull,
So it's very hard to break it.*

*When my head was shaken hard,
my brain sloshed to and fro.
It bounced within its tiny case,
Having no place else to go.*

*I never liked those jellyfish.
Yet I let my brain accrue one.
It's not white or red. It's worse.
It's probably a "blue" one.*

CHAPTER ELEVEN

THE FINAL STRAW

In May, as the trees started to fill out and the flowers began to sprout through the ground, I felt a little more adventurous. It was time I tried my "wings" and ventured forth out of Maine, doing my own thing alone.

I planned a trip to Boston to volunteer to help at the Level 10 National Gymnastics Championships. It would provide me with the opportunity to work independently for a change. I would be assigned duties to assist the running of the meet in any way needed. I was a little hesitant, as I didn't know the specific tasks I would be doing until I arrived, and I would be staying by myself in the hotel.

I had not driven in the city yet, or traveled to any place where I needed to follow directions alone, while driving. If I felt any doubt that I could do it, I never let anyone else know, for fear that the trip would be put on hold until I gained more experience. I asked for assurances and directions from people within the rehabilitation hospital, who I knew cared about me, but wouldn't be overly concerned. Then I assured Gordon that I could take care of everything.

I left with packed suitcases, a sureness that I was fine, and written directions on which exits to use. I had been to Boston on many previous occasions and did not harbor any doubts or foresee any problems that I might not be able to handle.

I arrived in Boston quite easily. After I exited from the main thoroughfare onto the side streets of the city, I started to look for anything that would lead me to the host hotel. As I maneuvered my car down one-way streets and looked up, I could see the bright red letters of the Sheraton, high on a building, somewhere to the left. It was behind a row of other buildings, but I could tell in what direction to go. I headed my car toward the direction of the sign. When I arrived where I thought the building should be, it wasn't there. Slowly I continued to move in and out of traffic, trying to get a glimpse over the buildings in order to try again. Needless to say, this scenario occurred many times. An hour and a half later, I was still going around in circles becoming more and more frustrated with each turn.

As I slowly headed down a narrow side street, I noticed a patrolman ahead. He had a familiar look about him. I slowed down, lowered my window and said, "Excuse me. Could you tell me how to get to the Sheraton?" He turned toward me and said "Damn it, lady. You've asked me THREE times already." I shrunk down in my seat, and listened carefully as he started telling me again. I didn't remember stopping, or asking, or his telling me ever before. I never questioned that he had, because he did have that air of familiarity about him that I couldn't explain. I found the hotel, which just goes to show that repetition really works.

The next morning when it was time to go to the arena, I took out the map sent to me by the gymnastics committee. Knowing the problem that I had finding the hotel, I had serious doubts that I would ever make the arena on time, even though it was less than a quarter of a mile away. I made a more practical decision and called a cab. The cost was added to an already expensive volunteer weekend, but it got me there.

Upon arriving I found the arena locked and empty. I had become so focused on the directions, that I had forgotten about going to breakfast and had arrived three hours early. So I sat down on a bench and waited.

Eventually people arrived and we were given our assignments. Mine was to work in the copy room and run the copies of the running scores for the meet personnel and press. It was a good job for me because I was familiar with copy machines. And I didn't have to be involved with the noise of the arena, crowds and gymnasts. But when I found the room that hac1d the copy machines, I saw thousands of program pages, stacked and waiting to be collated and assembled. That mass project was obviously going to take place in the same room.

I worked on covers, cutting, stapling, assembling and every hour or so helped a new crew learn how to assemble the programs. I didn't break for lunch or dinner. In fact, I never left the room. It was 9:30 P.M. before I had finished running the final meet results for the day. I was one of the last people to leave, using a phone in the lobby to call a cab. When I arrived back at the hotel, I realized that I had passed the point of my ability to cope. Tomorrow would bring more of the same, and I could not handle the confusion. I was exhausted and I decided to go home RIGHT NOW. I knew that someone else would take over the job on the next day, and with so many people working, I would never even be missed.

But first, I had to call Gordon and tell him that I was leaving for home. When he answered the phone (well after 11 P.M.) and heard my frustration and confusion, he knew how tired I was. He agreed that coming home was a very good idea...just not at that time, and definitely not in the condition I was obviously in. I screamed over the phone at him. "What condition?" He calmly said, "You're too tired to drive tonight, Bev." He suggested that I go to my room and get a good night's sleep first.

I had been told to go to my room many times as a patient early in recovery, when I got over-stimulated, and I drew a comparison between then and now. He was probably right. I would have to pay for my room anyway. I would start home in the morning more refreshed. Although I had a tremendous urge to get out of there immediately, I went to my room and reluctantly settled in for the night.

In the morning I was tempted to repeat the experience of the day before. But I decided to stay with my decision. As I left the hotel, I passed hordes of gymnasts in the lobby, waiting to be transported to the arena. I could only think of herds of sheep being led to the slaughter...an odd thought for a sport I loved so much. I gave silent thanks to God that I was going in the other direction for a change.

As I exited the city after a few wrong turns, I felt a tremendous surge of relief. I also felt the pangs of guilt. For the first time in my career or that I could ever remember, I had not lived up to a commitment I had made. I felt a little better knowing it was for the best, but there was still a part of me that hurt. Maybe it was the first time that I actually realized that I had to take care of ME.

It would be a more peaceful ride home. I turned on the cassette player and quickly became "one" with my music. After about ten miles or so, I noticed my cruise control settings on my wheel. I wondered if I could remember how to put on the cruise control. I was pleased when the car took off at a steady 68 miles an hour, and I had to do nothing.

I folded my feet under me and thought of all the things that were waiting for me to do at home, ones that didn't require noise, crowds, confusion and overload.

It was a three lane highway. As I passed some cars, I changed lanes both to the right and left. After about ten miles, the traffic slowed and started to get a little heavier. Instead of passing one car at a time, I began to pass cars that were two abreast of each other. I rapidly approached cars that were traveling slower than I was. As I weaved in and out, between lanes, I suddenly wondered what on earth I would do if I came to THREE cars abreast of each other. I couldn't pass them, because there were only three lanes. How was I supposed to get around them? How would I let them know my car was coming by and it was on automatic pilot. I became very concerned. I knew there was an answer, but what it was, I couldn't figure out. Other drivers must have run into this same problem and my mind became frantically engrossed with trying to find a solution. My eyes watched warily ahead for the three cars abreast, that would mean my nemesis. I not only had no idea of how to shut the cruise control off, but even more frightening, the possibility never even occurred to me. I was only concerned with how I would pass these three cars, when I came up behind them.

At some point I must have touched the brake, because the cruise control eventually went off. Miles later, while trying to figure out what happened, I made a decision not to use my cruise control again.

Whatever "automatic behavior" should have occurred, didn't. Something in my brain had shut off and I had not been functioning correctly. Slowly, I became aware of the danger of what had happened. I not only didn't decipher the solution, I didn't even have a clue to the real problem.

This time I had improved a bit though. I did recognize that something had just happened that shouldn't have. I must take steps to see that my body, not the car, is always on automatic pilot and knows what to do. My inability to know what to do actually frightened me, the more I thought about it. I drove slower the rest of the way home.

I shared my experiences with Gordon. We talked about all of them. I wasn't sure which was the most discouraging. But I had learned that I still 1had a ways to go, and that I needed to avoid so much stress and confusion in the future.

I, also, shared my experience with the cruise control with Dr. Marks that week. He reiterated patiently, about my difficulty with initiation because of frontal lobe dysfunction and how it was all related.

Even more important, he reemphasized how I had to be careful. That was easier said than done. But he didn't need to worry. I had already decided to never use my cruise control again.

Dr. Marks and I worked together to see that my driving became as safe as it could be. He went for rides with me in the car to make sure that I was using the strategies we talked about. It also gave him a chance to spot other problems I might be having.

I drove him through the city and over the back roads to the ocean. We inevitably ended up at the lighthouse. We both enjoyed lighthouses. There was always something about them that was soothing to me. They seemed to be able to put the unknown endings in my life in proper perspective. I think it is the old eternal circling that symbolizes that "What Goes Around, Comes Around", philosophy of life.

We took a moment or two to stand and watch the sea before heading back over the road to the hospital again. I think he felt better about my driving, knowing I was safe. I know I felt better, thinking he felt safer about my driving.

In any case, I grew to trust Dr. Marks and his ability to help my driving skills. He dealt with me honestly, as together we invented new and different strategies that would work for me. I would implement them and he would tell me if they were doing what I needed to have done.

Thanks to him, my recovery did not stop with just being on the road again. He worked diligently and delicately with me to keep me, and others, safe. I know there were times that were scary, and times that we both held our breath. But without those times, I would never have been able to compensate for the vast deficits that I had to deal with.

Those people who predicted I would never drive again were wrong. They didn't know me. They didn't know the determination that lies within this person. Neither did they realize what strength there is in teamwork, when solutions need to be found.

Dr. Marks brought me from a state of unawareness to a state of independence on the road. It was not an easy journey and at times it was a very frightening one. But without his help and guidance, I would not be behind the wheel today. I know that is a fact.

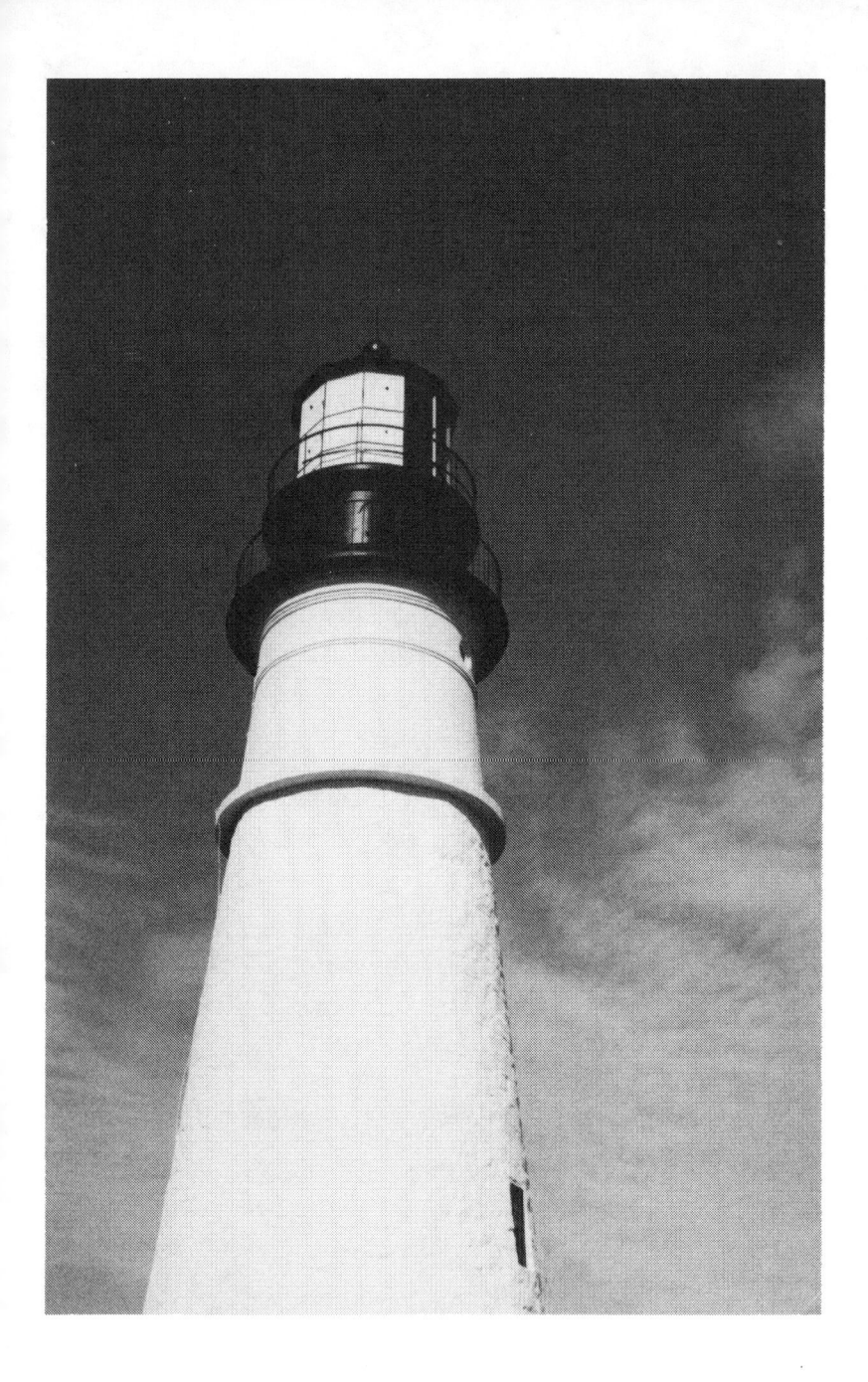

A LIGHTHOUSE

*There is a beacon out there
Just beyond my reach,
Sending its moving beam of light
Slicing through the fog
Blackness, then light,
Then blackness again.*

*I watch it, fascinated as it circles,
Revolving and approaching,
Retreating and advancing,
Taking its time arriving, yet
Leaving just as surely as it comes.*

*I wonder if it touches more out there,
And if it does, where its journey ends.
Sometimes, even where it begins in the
Light, then blackness
Then light again.*

*The silence broken only by the loud,
Low honking of the horn,
From somewhere far beyond,
Calling to wanderers
Lost within the blackness
Trying to find their way home.*

*One beacon, standing alone,
Guarding against collision
By the only way it knows.*

SECTION FOUR

TOWARD NEW HORIZONS

CHAPTER TWELVE

THE BOOK

Evenings when George, my computer job coach, wasn't assigned to work with me, I started to work on the book. It was my own project, and would be done without any assistance from other people, especially professionals. They had provided the material for the book by dealing and working with me, but I was going to show them that I was able to think for myself, and able to understand more than anyone really believed I could. They should learn, too, to expect more from the patients and clients they treat, and not set limits for persons with brain injury. With people without injury, you never know their capabilities until they are challenged. I wanted professionals who deal with brain injury survivors to know that they should never limit their expectations either. One never knows other people's limits.

Sometimes an idea that can be brought to fruition through creative means, can be worth much more than the money it takes to do it. I decided then, that not only would I write a book, but I would attempt to have it return some real value to the brain injury community, for professionals, survivors and their families. So I would make sure that what I recorded was accurate, meaningful and would make a difference.

In order to do that, I knew I would have to share intimate moments, experiences, thoughts and feelings that were still locked within me. I would find a way when the time came. I knew that writing the book would be the easiest part for me. Sharing it would be the hardest. I didn't know if I could do that. I would wait and think about that when I had finished. My goal now, was to prove I could write it.

We are all unique individuals and need to be challenged and allowed to set and reach our own goals. And if we fail, we will have learned hopefully, to set new goals and try again. Without that challenge and growth, it is hard to develop a real sense of worth. I had learned already that I was entitled to the right to succeed. In order to do that, I must also be allowed the right to fail in the attempt.

*"There are no such things as failures,
only successes that grow out of them."*

The first thing that I knew I had to do to begin my book and start on my adventure was to get accurate information. Since my memory was severely impaired, I had to see everything at once in one place to grasp it. I went to the rehabilitation hospital and asked my physicians to allow me to study my medical records. They let me see them and copy whatever I needed. With these notes and my memory book, that I kept every day as an inpatient and outpatient, I would have an accurate record of what transpired. By recording the information from my medical records and from my memory notebook into the computer, I would have a visible progression of my recovery.

The second step was to devise a way to handle all the information and to organize it into amounts I could process. My speech therapist had drummed into my head, that if I was to succeed with large tasks, that I had to break them down into smaller ones that I could handle.

So I made my first book writing strategy. I would have to write the book in chronological order. That would set limits on each chapter and keep me focused on one specific time frame and one topic at a time. I tried to make each incident into a separate chapter, so that I could study it in detail.

What I discovered was that I couldn't stay focused on any one thing for very long. As I read in my notes about things that happened, it would remind me about other things and I would get distracted. The feelings that I had experienced, came out as poetry. I never had to stop and think about them. They just flowed out of my head as entities.

Sometimes when I was reading of incidents recorded by the nurses, it would trigger other memories or feelings. I would ask someone else who was there at the time the incident happened, and they would remember it too. Slowly I could repiece incidents and feelings. As I read about certain events, I remembered my feelings about them more often than the events themselves. I faithfully recorded those feelings.

My book was actually written by using my deficits as strengths. Each morning my husband would literally lead me into the den, sit me down in front of my computer, turn it on and see that my writing program was on the screen. (That was the only program I could use.) He would place my C.D. earphones on my ears, turn on the lamp over the computer, turn the telephone ringer volume down and put on the answering machine. Then once I had begun to write, he would leave and close the den door. I would continue to write without stopping, until he came home for lunch. He would come in at noon, take off my earphones and tell me it was time for lunch. We would make lunch together and then we would repeat the process. Only in the afternoon, he had learned to shut the shades.

One afternoon, before he realized he had to close the curtains, I was distracted by the mailman driving by, and got up to get the mail. But by the time I got to the mailbox, the mail truck was further down the street. I failed to comprehend that the mail was already in the mailbox, and followed the truck down the street. Luckily Gordon came home and retrieved me from my journey.

We learned by the errors I made and changed our procedures to eliminate them. Once I started writing, I never rose from the chair until Gordon returned. I never went to the bathroom or anything. He left a drink for me and if I got tired while writing, I fell asleep in the chair. When I awoke, I found myself looking at the computer and just continued typing away.

Whether it was perseverance or perseveration, only professionals know. But it worked. Many times I stayed in the chair for 12 to 16 hours at a stretch. The book took four months to write. The hardest parts were the beginning and the ending. I never thought I would end it. I had no problems with each part or page, but trying to keep a continuous flow to the book was hard. Seeing the book as a whole entity was impossible for me, so I tried to concentrate on each part individually.

I learned as I wrote. I began to see the progress as it happened, that I couldn't see while I was undergoing it. I found myself learning about brain injury from myself.

I never told anyone how I managed to stay on task. It was embarrassing to admit the daily procedure we followed. But when you are on a roll, you keep throwing the dice. Take what works and use it.

No one really knows all of the possible ways to achieve success, but making progress means using every avenue, every strategy, every accommodation, and every way you can think of, to come out a winner. And I planned to be a winner. Pam was going to get to "eat my book".

Slowly my manuscript began to take shape. I don't think I ever had a total grasp of the whole thing at any one time. I know I hoped and prayed that the chapters would flow and continue without a break. I worked on the end of one chapter and the beginning of the next one at the same time, to try to connect them. I constantly had to go back to the beginning of the topic to reread what I had done as I would forget it as soon as it was written. I blessed the computer and the people who invented it. Without the computer, the task would have been impossible.

By late winter, the manuscript was ready to be shown to my very close friends to get a feeling of how it was. Was it interesting enough to hold your attention? Was it an accurate portrayal of what happened? I wanted to be sure my book was valid, too.

I wanted to share it first with Donna Levesque. She had been the one to first suggest that I write a book. She had planted the initial seed. I knew that she always had faith that I could do anything I tried, so I took it to her first.

For months, people within the hospital had

been asking me about the book. When I first started writing, I told people who inquired as to how I was doing, that I was writing a book. They just sort of nonchalantly nodded their heads. (Like, sure you are!) After all no one expects brain injury survivors to be able to do more than those who guide them. Each week they would ask me how far I had gotten, and each week I would tell them and they would ceremoniously nod again.

Everyone was interested in my progress, but some doubted that there was any book at all. Those who didn't, had no idea of the quality of book that was being finished. When I walked in with the manuscript and laid it on the CEO's desk, he was shocked to say the least. The comments were "We had no idea.." I can't really blame them. I didn't have any idea either.

The nurses on the head injury unit and the therapists I worked with, corroborated the events in the book. I felt satisfied. I never had any plans to go any further with the book. I had written it, and that was all I had planned to do. That had been the goal that I had taken on, to write a book. That was the challenge that I felt I had met.

After reading the manuscript, my friends insisted I should publish this book, and professionals told me that it would be very useful for others. Publishing it was not part of the original plan and I felt my job was done.

I proved my point and satisfied myself by writing the book that people said wasn't a realistic goal. Actually I was tired and not excited about another challenge. I wanted to present the manuscript to Pam and rest for a while.

Then one afternoon, a nurse who had read one of the incidences recorded in the book (and who had been on the scene when it had occurred), came and confided how much she had learned from hearing my perspective of what happened that day. She said she would never have looked at the incident from the way I was perceiving it. She told me how much she had learned from looking at things from my perspective. It was of great value to her in her work. Her sincerity impressed me. She made me stop and wonder if publishing the manuscript would be of value to other survivors, who couldn't express themselves the way I was able to do.

Should I or shouldn't I? Would I or wouldn't I? Decisions, decisions... I had so much trouble making decisions, even the easiest of them.

DECISIONS

Is it left or is it right?
Is it dull or is it bright?
Is it North or is it South?
Is it "ear" or is it "mouth"?

Will it be pork, beef or fish?
Will it be first or second wish?
Will it be light before it's dark?
Will it be here or in the park?

Is this for here or packed to go?
Is it secret or must they know?
Is it real or just a trial?
Is it remote or run by dial?

Will you be back again today?
Should I go or should I stay?
Does he love or does he not?
Did he not care or just forgot?

Was it Mickie D's or Burger King,
The King of Swat or the King of Swing?
Decisions! Decisions! I cannot take them.
I hate them all, 'cause I just can't make them.

I thought long and hard about the possibility of publishing my book. There were pros and cons on both sides. The publishing realm was a "dog eat dog" world and I was extremely unknowledgable, naive, and vulnerable. I really was unaware of the value of what I had written.

Although my book was conceived in anger, and finished in determination, it had been written in innocence. I only knew what had happened to me, and thought I was alone in my particular experience. I knew little about the multitudes of other head injury survivors out there.

I didn't really think anyone would want to read about some obscure accident to a person in Maine. I think the challenge of seeing if I could complete the task became a personal goal I had set for myself.

But what good was being able to write a book and doing it, if no one ever read it. So I made a decision. I would give it a try. I felt I had nothing to lose.

"I will do it all myself,
As I have done in long days past.
If the project gets too hard,
I'll know I stepped too far, too fast."

I hired a graphics arts designer to help me with the layout of the book in its final form, and a photographer who supplied pictures for several pages. I picked out a cover from a photograph taken by a local woman and my book started to take shape. We toured a local printing company and decided to have the book printed and bound there.

Now I only needed the funds to do it. It was about three weeks later, when a good friend mentioned to me confidentially that she would like to invest in some risky projects, just for the experience. I felt God had played a part.

I offered her a percentage of the net returns, if she not only funded part of the expenses, but physically helped me market it. I knew that would be hard for me to do without help. She quickly agreed. My book was underway. I was thrilled and, yet at the same time, felt afraid. Suddenly I had something very important to lose.

Revelation

*Should I seek to give away
What other people cannot see?
What is burrowed deep inside
That very private part of me?*

*For if I do, the world will know,
And part of me is gone for good.
I not only wonder if I dare,
But even more, If I should.*

Several times I started to call the printer to tell them to stop the presses. I didn't want to share that intimate part of me with the whole world. I wasn't sure that even if I wanted to, that I could. What I had written was very private, personal thoughts, emotions and feelings. Now they would no longer be mine alone. I wasn't sure that I wanted that loss either.

Everyone would know my weaknesses and I didn't want any sympathy, I needed strength. Perhaps it was good to write the book to release these feelings and anger, but letting the whole world see them, was not part of the original bargain.

"Beverley, What were you ever thinking?"

I never got around to initiating the "stop action" and six weeks later, 3000 copies of my books rolled off the presses.

The printer called and asked me to be there to check out the colors on the covers as they were being printed. What a feeling when I suddenly saw the covers and title staring up at me from the bottom of the presses. Shivers went through me as I realized I had actually done it. I had proved that people with brain injury are capable of creating and meeting goals, if they are willing to put in the effort. Some people's goals might not be this complex, but all persons with brain injury have their individual goals to aim for. People who work with them must believe in them too.

So my book, IN SEARCH OF WINGS, became a reality through determination. Oh! I made some mistakes. I will not make the same mistakes again, because I took the time to write them all down. It was a very good learning experience, and I need to take advantage of every lesson.

I also knew that I had reached the point of no return, and my decision to be silent no more would have ramifications for me very soon.

SURVIVOR'S VOICE

*I've made a choice
that I knew I must make.
And traveled a journey
that no one should take.
My brain has been injured
through no fault of mine.
I've spent too long searching
for reasons to find
out, why it was me?
But that doesn't matter.
I've not spoken out
and that's even sadder.*

*I thought what was happening
should be hidden, you see.
I never knew millions
were struggling like me.
Now I know who I am
and demand recognition.
I'm a capable person
and invite competition.
I'm working through days
and long into the nights,
to declare and retrieve
my God-given rights.
I may never again be
who I was before.
But I promise you this,
I'll be silent no more!*

CHAPTER THIRTEEN

REDESIGNING DESTINATIONS

The first copy of my book went to Pam, my vocational rehabilitation counselor. I told her it was for dessert. She was shocked, but very impressed and pleased. I understand why she was surprised. I do write better than I appear to function, because the computer becomes my "brain" and allows me to remember what would otherwise be forgotten, before I can get it down on paper. God bless computers for brain injury rehabilitation. Pam said she learned to set higher expectations for her clients. I felt proud.

After Pam read my book, my VR program became one designed by me. I was given the opportunity to change and plan my own goals and Pam became a supporter in my efforts. We worked together to develop a very realistic program that was geared to assist me in becoming independent in work situations. I tried hard, knowing that nothing worth doing is ever easy. We work well together as a team.

My Individualized Written Rehab Plan is now my own. I revised and wrote it myself. I was going to work toward three new goals that would challenge me to become, not only independent in the work force, but hopefully, my work would help others become motivated to become more independent as well.

GOAL ONE

My first new goal was to continue to work toward becoming independent with my computer for the rental business. While I had made much progress with my bookkeeping program, it was obvious that I would never be able to achieve total independence with the program I was currently using. So my team met and made the recomnmendation that I be scheduled for updated neuropsychological testing to ascertain my present strengths and weaknesses. My last one had been almost two years ago, and I obviously had recovered a lot since then. Hopefully this testing would guide the team in developing my vocational program to accommodate these new changes.

So I underwent another round of tests to determine the extent of improvement over the past two years. My last testing had been done after I was discharged from New England Rehabilitation Hospital as an inpatient. Hopefully we would find out how we could best utilize my computer to compensate for what I had trouble doing. Dr. Marks let me know that he was concerned about retesting me. He said that many of the things that I relearned to do, were the result of super-compensatory strategies. These would be negated because during testing, I could not rely on these strategies. The testing did not measure my ability to use them. He did not want me to get discouraged, if the test did not show improvement. He'd be surprised if there was any organic functioning change. If I was willing to accept that, he would schedule testing.

That was all right with me. I knew my limits. I also knew that parts of my brain were working much faster than a couple of years before. Sometimes, in fact, my brain went so fast, I couldn't keep up with the processing. Images and thoughts went so fast, I couldn't shut them out.

During those time, I needed to rest, with no stimulation or play my music at an incredible volume to shut down the processing. Other times, I needed very soft music to relax. When my brain went into super-mode, I needed to over-ride it manually. There were things, I was sure, that had not improved, but if I could deal with them in real life and compensate for them, they did not concern me.

I was pleased with the results of my testing. I felt Dr. Marks was also very surprised.

During college my I.Q. had ranged in testing from 146 - 158. In 1991, at my last testing, I registered at 110. I knew that I had undergone a tremendous loss at that time, but no one else did. After all, my scores were still in the high average range. But I couldn't pay attention, process or remember. Now I tested out at 135. I had learned not to think when people asked me a question that required calculation. The answers were in my head immediately, but if I thought, even for a moment, before answering, I forgot the question and the answer. Then I never got ready for the next question. So I was able to work faster now, by not taking the time to organize answers, think about procedures, or to visually compute problems. If I just reeled off the answer that came into my head without thinking, it was usually right. This is what I would have done preinjury.

Unfortunately, my attempt to do that in real life situations was the part that had gotten me into real trouble. I had been very thoroughly indoctrinated into the importance of not saying or doing anything without thinking, in order to curb my impulsivity.

My selected, sustained and divided attention skills were impaired. I knew that, but using strategies enabled me to be quite functional in those areas. My problem with my computer was in these areas. I had other problems in my life because of these deficits, but we had been working on them in functional situations since my injury and I felt we had been very successful.

My biggest disappointment was in my memory. The tests showed that I still had severe deficits in both visual and verbal memory. I really thought that had improved. It was obvious now that it had only seemed so, because I had been so diligent in using my memory notebook and writing down my life. What I thought had been restorative, had only been achieved through compensatory strategies. But that, also, explained why I could never remember things, even when I really exerted effort to apply myself, focusing in and paying close attention.

Dr. Marks was very pleased with the testing results. He said I showed much more improvement than he had expected, especially in some of the attention areas, in tracking, and my ability to not get distracted in close settings. He said my brain showed organic improvement in the frontal areas. This was unusual after so much time.

He felt the testing was valuable in helping him devise a computer program for me that would be meaningful and would meet my specific needs. He suggested VR have a program written that would use only my strengths.

So a new plan was developed to have a more user-friendly program designed especially for me to compensate for my severe memory and attentional deficits. An original individualized program was to be written that was menu-driven and could be initiated totally from the monitor. This new program would allow me to keep my eyes on the screen and find information needed in the windows.

It was a long process to begin over again, but progress toward becoming independent, as we knew, had many curves. A successful program always evaluates what works and changes what doesn't. We needed to change course to see that I regained the ability to work independently.

Scott Jacobson, a computer programmer, was hired on the team to write my program. Dr. Marks worked with him closely to see that this new program met all of my special needs, and that I was able to do what the program needed to have done. The team that worked closely together consisted of Pam Williams, my state VR Counselor; David Marks, my neuropsychologist; KoKo Keller, my on-site rehab counselor (who I'll discuss later); my husband, Gordon; my job coach, George who understood the program that we used now; and me. I knew it might take a while, but returning me to independencce was the ultimate goal that I was ready to work for, and my team was too. My team was a great one.

It was survivor-driven. I was their main concern and my needs became all important. We had to learn to work together for my best interests. My job was to stay motivated and determined and, believe me, I tried.

It took about 5 months to write the program, and teach it to me so that I could understand it and operate it alone. The goal was to install it in my home on my computer and be in use for the first of the year.

I trained at Scott's home on his computer for about 3 1/2 months. He lived near the hospital and it was easier to work there. He could make changes as they were needed and correct the glitches that kept popping up. The program needed to be complex enough to do all the necessary work, yet easy enough to self-cue me as to the next step. We used colors, signs, positions, markers, and sizing for cues.

My husband, Gordon, knew nothing about computers, and cared to know even less. He even became excited about the new program. He could understand it too. This was necessary because he would eventually become the one to work with me, after Scott left.

I learned by sitting at Scott's computer and entering transactions he made up. He would sit behind me with a laptop computer. When I floundered, he would ask me what was wrong. I would say "I can't find the FIND button." He would tell me it was in the upper right corner. Then when I stalled again, he would ask again what was the matter? I would say, "I don't know what to do next." He would say, "Push TAB".

The next day when I came back, the FIND button would be painted hot pink, and where I got lost and didn't know what to do, on the screen would be printed PUSH TAB. That was how we worked. He was wonderful with creative techniques in working with people who are physically or mentally challenged.

When January arrived, the program was

installed on our computer at home and I was entering transactions on my own. I started doing just the transactions. Then within three months I was printing my monthly reports by myself. Scott became only a phone call away if I needed him.

As I became more familiar with the routine of what I was doing, I gradually started reading the sections of the computer tutorial that explained different things. I can't say that I remember much, but it sometimes enabled me to solve immediate problems on my own.

In July we revamped and revised the program so that the six month reports were similar and contained the same information that I would need for income tax purposes in December. From that time on, I was working on my own. Scott was on long-term support, just in case.

This whole process has taken two years. It has been a hard and busy two years. It required a lot of effort on my part to stay interested and excited and not to slack off when I got tired.

Enabling me to become independent in my business was a total team effort. I provided the motivation, effort and desire. VR provided the knowledge, funding, and help. I felt a renewed feeling of self-worth, because my team saw that changes were needed and made them. Making changes is hard...hard for programs, pocketbooks, counselors, and most of all, clients. But the ability to change and adapt and the willingness to do so, are the vital links to success.

Pam is a wonderful VR counselor to have in my corner. She is a learner. They are the best kind, the kind that are always looking out for the best interests of their clients and is willing to admit that they, also, learn in the process. They are the rare ones that state agencies find hard to keep on the payroll, and clients with brain injury don't usually get. I like Pam very much. I only hoped she never leaves, not only because of her expertise, but because brain injury survivors don't deal with changing therapists or counselors very well.

Either Maine Vocational Rehabilitation has very special people working for them, or I was extremely fortunate to get the best. I'd like to think both are true.

There comes a time when

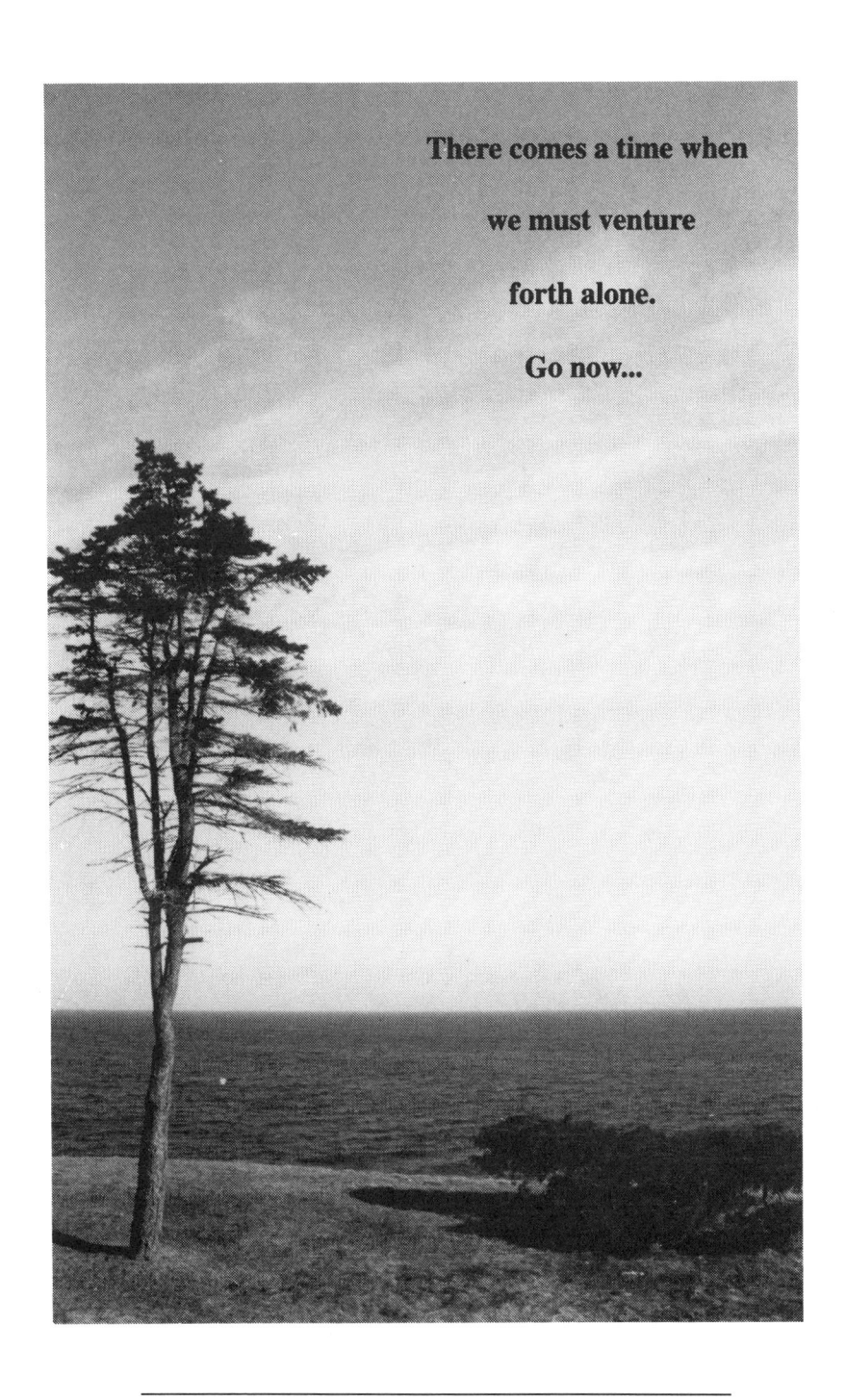

we must venture

forth alone.

Go now...

SECTION FIVE

IMPRINTS

CHAPTER FOURTEEN

FROM CARRIE'S PERSPECTIVE

I was 24 years old when Mom had her accident. I was living on my own in an apartment in South Paris. Being single, I had daily exposure to Mom after her injury. I had graduated from the University of Maine in Child Development and was in the middle of my third year of teaching at the Hartford-Sumner Elementary School.

My father called me the following morning and said Mom had been in a car accident. She was okay, seemed to have a concussion, but they had admitted her to the hospital.

When I visited her I was relieved that she didn't appear more seriously injured. All of us laughed, when the staff told us that she had told the *emergency room doctors that her husband's name was John. I was worried about her, because she was very confused, had trouble walking and yet, insisted on getting out of bed. My life went from day to day, never knowing what was happening. When she left the hospital in February, I thought she was cured.*

She kept all of the things she had trouble doing, to herself. I did notice that when I talked to her, she would drift off and not seem interested in what I was saying. She had difficulty following any conversation. This happened after only a few sentences, whenever I tried to tell her something. She would become disinterested and I would become frustrated with her. After all, she had always been my best listener. Unaware that she was not able to stay tuned in, I felt she was no longer interested in me.

When I asked her to help me make decisions, and she couldn't, I was hurt. Little did I realize, she couldn't make decisions anymore for herself. When I asked her for advice, which she was always good at giving before, she just sat there mesmerized, unable to help.

Looking back, it was in these subtle ways that my mother had changed. I thought she was just too busy and never, for a moment, related her actions to the accident.

When she re-entered the hospital in July, I knew it was much more serious. The family was drastically worried, and the doctors didn't know what to expect. She couldn't use her right arm or her right leg. She didn't talk much, so I suspected that she was confused, and didn't want us to know.

In time, she was allowed to get out of bed using a walker. The nurses would tell me how she wandered unsupervised, and then couldn't find her room again.

I became upset with her for making the nurses worry. But mom didn't remember what she did. I didn't understand what was happening. My mother would never purposely worry anyone. She cherished being in charge of her own life.

When the decision was made to send her to New England Rehabilitation Hospital, I felt very guilty. I knew that our family doctor had told Mom before, that a rehabilitation hospital was a place she'd never want to be. I felt guilty that now we were sending her to one, and I couldn't stop it.

One day when I visited her, she went to speech therapy. I found myself listening at the door. Even though the therapist had invited me in to observe the session, I chose to listen outside the door alone. The therapist talked to my mother slowly, like she was a child. I wanted to go right in, and tell this woman how incredibly smart my mother was. What a great memory she had, and how she didn't need to be talked to like my students. But then, I noticed my mother was answering her slowly, too. She wasn't answering some of the easy questions that my first graders would have known. This wasn't like her, and I didn't understand . She always knew the answers to everything. I couldn't believe that my mother had changed so much, and I didn't see it.

The staff insisted that Mom be "grey-belted" for safety reasons. I never dreamed that anyone would ever feel that my Mom needed to be restrained. Many times, when I came to visit, she would ask me to take off the belt. She told me calmly that she didn't need it, and would not get out of the wheelchair. I felt sorry for her, and didn't have any reason not to trust her, so I would take it off. It was a while before I learned that when I left her after visiting hours, she would impulsively rise out of her chair without locking it, and and head for places unknown. I did not believe others, when they told me of my mother's exploits throughout the hospital. I knew my mother better than they did.

I was confused as to what was really happening. Part of me still didn't understand why she was still at the hospital after so many weeks. She kept telling everyone she was fine.

While at work, I found myself in tears, whenever anyone asked me how she was doing, because I couldn't explain what was wrong with her. I had never heard of traumatic brain injury and never expected my own mother to become a victim.

After Mom had been there for about two

I was allowed to take her to the Maine Mall on a shopping trip during a day pass. We had not gone more than 200 feet in my car, when another car pulled in front of us without signaling. As I yelled and jammed on the brakes, my mother calmly and quickly gave the man "the finger". Not a quick up and down gesture, but a constant one in the window. She did not seem to know or care about what she had done. I was infuriated. I spoke to her like she was a child. I yelled at her to SIT on her hands. I suddenly knew that my Mom had changed. She would never even use a swear word. While we were growing up, she insisted that we use proper English and act with dignity wherever we went. Something was very wrong.

The family conferences that were held, and there were several, seemed to be one way. More for the staff to interact and discuss Mom's status. We seemed rushed during the 30 minute allottment. It often took 10 minutes or so, just to have all the staff arrive and to get a room, and there was always some therapist or doctor who had to leave early, or couldn't come at all. Questions we wanted to ask seemed an imposition on somebody's time. It was also hard to ask questions with my Mom present. The staff talked in terms of what they were doing for her in therapy, but they never explained to us exactly what was wrong with her. So even though there were conferences, they were for the most part, not as informative or as valuable as I wished they had been.

I learned eventually what was really

happening from the nursing staff, who worked with her, and dealt with her, and chased her all day. They explained to me what brain injury was all about and that Mom was doing exactly what persons with brain injury do. They described the progress she was making. When I finally admitted to myself that something was drastically wrong with my mother, I felt even more guilty that I had not recognized it earlier.

When she came home, it was obvious that she had changed. She was quiet and didn't talk much. She didn't admit her deficits and, as always, tried to do everything herself. I trusted her, and even then, I still didn't knkow that she could not be relied upon to do what she said. She meant well, but would forget what she said and do whatever popped into her mind.

So while I had to deal with the person who looked like my mother, but acted like someone I didn't know, my biggest loss was my best friend. We had always been best of friends, as well as mother and daughter. Now the roles were reversed. I found myself taking care of her. I was responsible for her, and no one was responsible for me.

Brain injury didn't just hurt my Mom. It hurt all of us. Being there and being involved made it even harder to deal with.

Mom's book IN SEARCH OF WINGS came out during her recovery. I had no idea of the kind of book she was busily writing. When she showed it to me, I laughed and I cried, but most of all, it has helped me to better understand brain injury and the difficulties one has to face. I learned more about brain injury from my own mother's book, than all the information I received during her recovery. Understanding the devastation of brain injury is hard enough, but living with it is a day-to-day challenge.

It's been four years since that day when I listened at the speech therapist's door. My mom had improved greatly since then. I have learned to recognize many of the things that she has had to overcome.

I still find myself learning new things about brain injury from being with her, and more often, forgetting the things that have changed between us. My mother is back to being my Mom and best friend again.

We do things a little differently than we did before. I still realize that my Mom can't stay tuned in to any lengthy conversations. If she is tired or stressed, she will get distracted, no matter how important what I am saying is. I keep my communication short. But I understand now that she still cares abaout my day and is trying her best to listen.

We take trips now, just for fun, to relax and get away. We go to the movies, theatre, and listen to music together. Perhaps, I have learned to become *more patient because of mom's injury. If so, I hope it rubs off in other areas of my life.*

Mom comes to my house for dinner and I go home several times a week. What I do find is that I am building a great relationship with my dad. since Mom has changed. I have recently bought my own home, and while Mom volunteers at the hospital, Dad has been able to spend time helping me make minor repairs. Mom, who previous to her accident, loved to decorate and remodel rooms, still has a difficult time making decisions on her own. So when it comes down to choosing colors to paint walls, or what to put where, I have to rely on my own decisions. Instead of asking for Mom's opinion on which choice to make, I decide myself and then share what I have decided with her. It allows her to realize that I still value her approval, and takes the pressure off her decision-making.

Sometimes, when we are together, I even forget that Mom is different now. When we talk, laugh, sing, take trips and reminesce, I am astounded at how much she is the same. She remembers things from the past with uncanny accuracy, often better than I. She still thinks of a thousand things at once, and tries to do them all.

I am only reminded of her limitations, when she can't remember the trip we just took yesterday, where we ate lunch today, or a telephone call she just took. It is then that I know I need to take a minute and try to cherish each moment with her, because it might be lost forever.

When she gets impatient, which she does, I try to be tolerant . I plan to be on time, because I know she has a hard time dealing with being late. She avoids conflict of any kind and so I try to shield her from anyproblems and stay calm when I am around her. Also, she has become much more aware of the impact of her injury on us. Because she decided to write a second book dealing with the continuing process, I am confident that we bridged a large gap in the recovery process. It also serves as a validation of our change as a family, and what we have experienced since her injury, and all of our attempts at dealing with it.

Even though I know that part of my mother has changed permanently , I also have come to realize the importance of accepting change and changing with it. We've learned to become more aware of feelings, rather than actions. We focus on how we are doing, rather than what we are doing.

Mom has not slowed down much. I doubt she ever will. She needs to be busy and productive. She just has to be more careful of her limitations now. I'm not sure she's come to grip with that yet.

Our family is much stronger today than ever before. Working as a unit, we are much more open about our feelings and needs. In spite of all of the changes, we have a very strong hope and determination in the future.

Last week, on my folks 33rd wedding anniversary, we went out deep sea fishing. Both of my parents love the ocean. On the way back into the harbor, my Mom decided to take pictures of the seagulls flying overhead. She had a film of 36 exposures and took the whole roll photographing the birds. I looked at Dad expecting him to suggest to her that she might have enough. If there were 100 exposures, she would probably take 100 pictures. Dad just watched, smiled and let her do her thing. Suddenly I smiled, too, as I remembered that those pictures would probably be her only memory of a very special day.

We still, and probably always will, feel as if we need to protect Mom. We love her, both as she was, and as she is. Dad doesn't allow anyone to set limits for Mom anymore. She makes her own.

I know she often feels she has the surge and power of oceans within her and needs to run with the tides. Sometimes just the soft current of a bubbling brook would be enough for me.

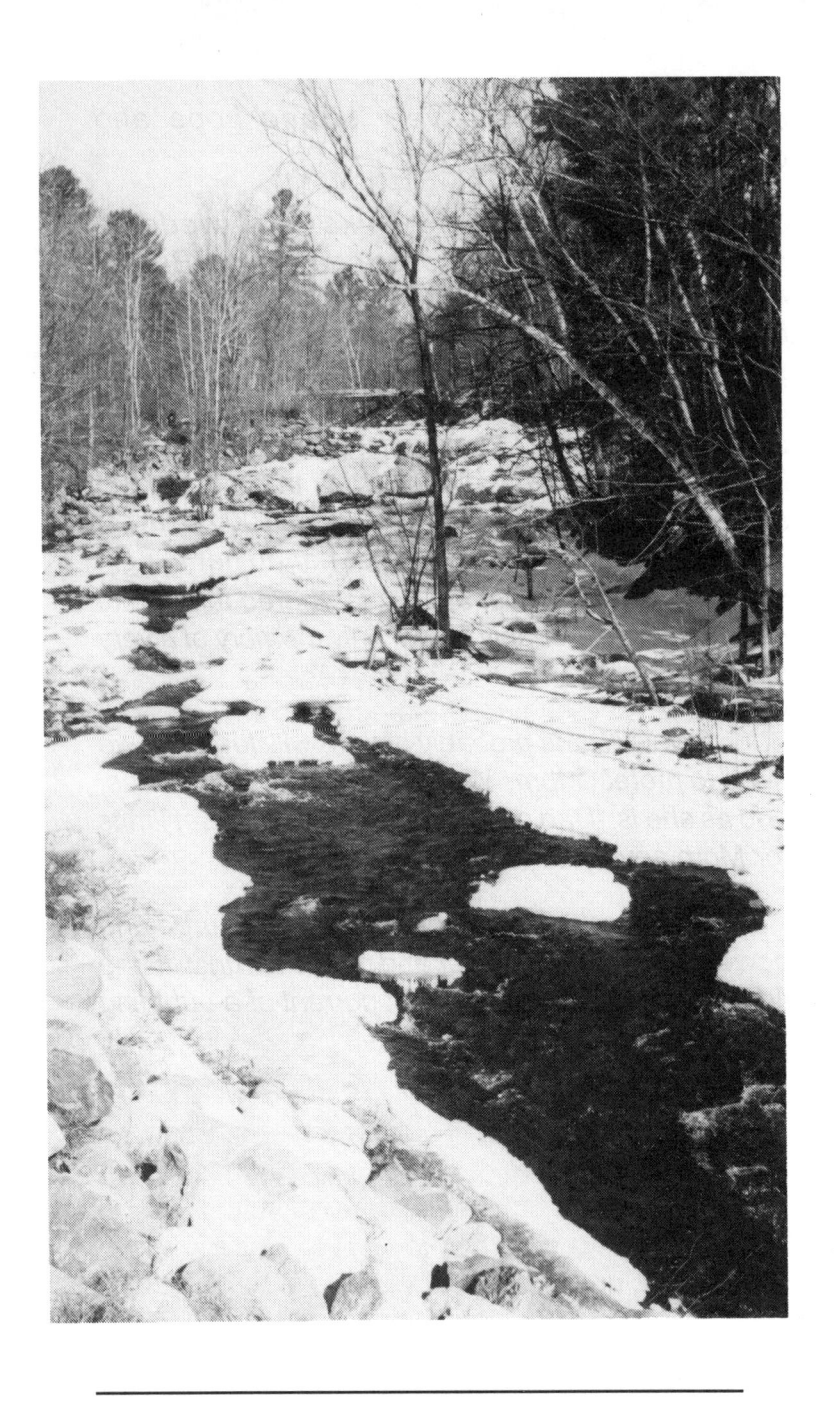

CHAPTER FIFTEEN

CHALLENGES- BOOK TWO

My second goal was to write another book, doing the layout and graphics completely myself, and to deal with the marketing of my first book. I wanted to write about my experience of returning to the road, the total vocational experience, and a family perspective.

Even though I had completely written IN SEARCH OF WINGS by myself, I felt that my unusual experiences in trying to return to driving should be shared with others. Maybe I could provide the opportunity for others to learn from my mistakes and my successes.

There is no skill in brain injury recovery that has more impact and danger than returning to driving. The desire to know if one can return to the road is a constant struggle in recovery. Maybe my experiences could illustrate the need to wait, and let it take as much time as possible. It might, also, make people aware that there are still deficits and problems that will not appear until after driving has reoccurred, and clients and professionals need to know of them.

I planned to complete this book from start to finish by myself. I had proved that I had the ability. I just had to be given the opportunity to use my organizational skills on a much higher level. This book would not be relegated to chronological order because of my deficits. I would deal with the whole experience in sections, rather than time. I didn't know if I could handle that. It was a more complicated task than ones I had already failed at before. Dealing with whole concepts at one time was still a large problem for me, but it would be a learning and challenging effort. One thing was for sure, I would give it my best attempt.

I planned to take courses and learn how to run the graphics, do the layout myself, and all the photography in the book would be mine. This book would be designed to meet financial goals suitable to vocational rehabilitation expectations.

So with Pam's blessing and George, my job coach assigned to go with me, I took a course to learn WordPerfect, a word processing program in our local adult education program. I soon learned that I was unable to learn in a classroom situation. I no longer learned by making mistakes. I could discover how to do things through trial and error, but once I got the right answer, I couldn't remember how I got there. I could learn something, only if I repeated it enough times in the same way. Taking the class and experimenting with different methods was not working. I had never been a quitter, but after five or six weeks of struggling, even with George beside me, I gave up the ghost. Discretion was the better part of valor. I had learned the hard way, to get myself out of situations that were not productive or were confusing for me. I was certain I could learn the program. I just had to find another path.

I knew if I did a task only the RIGHT way, and by repeating that right way over and over, hundreds of times, I would gradually learn. I was successful at some parts of it, by using the program in my volunteering work at the hospital. I recopied the Pharmacy's Policy and Procedure Manual from cover to cover and put it on a disk. It took me about four months, but I used Wordperfect. Those things I retained well, were through repetition of the same format over and over.

I took a course in graphics to see if I could learn Aldus Pagemaker program. I wanted to use that program to lay out the pages of my book. It was very difficult and I had to develop original ways to figure it out. I signed up for a practical graphics course using Pagemaker. The only problem was that I had an IBM and the course was on a Mac. It turned out to be BIG problem. George again tried to help me, but he was trying to learn it at the same time I was. I again found I did not learn by experimenting. I came away more discouraged about my ability to learn new information. Even with a job coach, I needed to have a very focused learning situation, or do things by rote and repetition. So we better utilized time by typesetting and printing.

By the end of the course, I made personalized pads of paper for Bryant Properties and Wings Publishing. It was a good experience and produced very useful products that I could use in my work. Hands on experience was good for me. I tended to remember better what I learned with my hands.

But more important, I was beginning to explore new arenas and take on challenges that tugged at my curiosity and made me excited about doing new things. I was beginning to lay down the parameters and understand the way in which I could be successful. Even more important, I was beginning to design my own plan of work.

I began the initial phase of laying out my outline for the book. It would be titled, TO WHEREVER OCEANS GO. I had been right in my assumptions. This one would be much harder for me to deal with, but there was no question that if given a chance, I could do it. I knew that driving and the support of vocational rehabilitaton were very important to other brain injury survivors and deserved special attention.

I didn't have many role models to follow, as I realized that not too many brain injury survivors were capable of taking on the complex challenges that I wanted and needed. But if I worked hard enough, I truly believed that I could become a role model for those survivors able to try. Maybe we could even create a path for others to follow, especially those who came to vocational rehabilitation with different needs than most.

I had heard horror stories from other survivors, both in my own and other states, who dealt with the system. I was sure that if people, survivors and professionals, only knew what was possible through working together, many of their problems would be made much easier. Maybe we all just need to evaluate our priorities every once in a while.

Survivors need to realize the importance of their work independence and counselors need to emphasize the importance of their client's needs and see that, whenever possible, they are met. I felt that my team was encouraging me to challenge myself.

Writing the second book was much harder than the first. I couldn't seem to put everything together. It involved family perspectives, and driving issues and vocational rehabiliation practices, plus it involved all of my jobs and roles that I was pursuing. Gymnastics, writing, driving, volunteering, support group facilitating, bookkeeping, counseling, brain injury work, public speaking were all areas in which I was intensely involved, and all of them were going on simultaneously. I couldn't seem to pull it all together. I worked for two years on writing the book, but I refused to give up.

When I finally felt that my book was ready for layout, I bought the software program, Aldus Pagemaker 5.0 and my husband made sure that I earned the money to pay for it myself. I had to earn it through speaking engagements and presentations. Once I had the program installed, I found I needed postscript language for the graphics. My printer would not do that. So I had to earn over $1000 to buy a new laser printer that would do the job. It took over 8 months of work to earn the money. Then once it was installed, I realized that I never learned how to use the program.

So two months later, which was only last week, I enrolled, without a job coach, at my own expense, in a college course in Pagemaker for Windows. This time it is geared to my needs. The course is being taught on IBM's in Windows. I lucked out. There are only five people in the course, so I am getting individual instruction.

I am following up with "Creative Design with Pagemaker", an advanced course, that will give me an opportunity to do the layout in class. Even though I chose not to finish the last course, I feel I have improved enough now to take what I can use, and ignore the rest. I take my work home and work on my assignments on my own computer. My book is beginning to take shape and I'm having a ball.

I am planning that TO WHEREVER OCEANS GO will be in the bookstores by spring. Once that is accomplished, there will be no limits for me pertaining to writing and publishing.

I'm psyched.

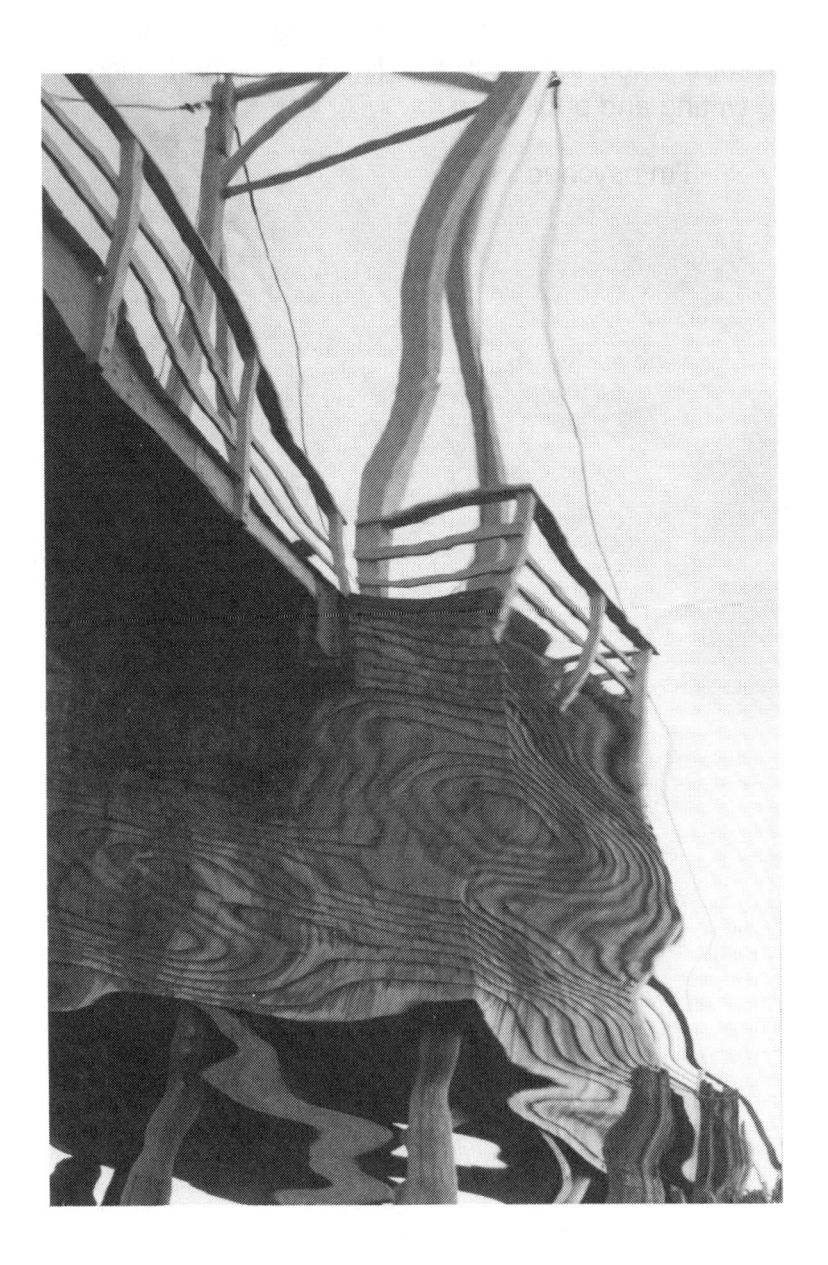

CHAPTER SIXTEEN

WHEN THE TIDE CHANGES, GO WITH THE CURRENT:

CHALLENGES FROM WITHIN

After I had been driving for about five months and doing well, I received the most stunning blow I could get. I was in the heights of my recovery. I had survived most of my deficits on the road and things were finally looking up. My first book was just ready to roll off the presses, and George and I were make progress with my bookkeeping skills. I was still relearning, at this time, the original program and was busily making tremendous progress. It was a time of excitement, and a time for celebration of my newly-recovered independence. But God, in his infinite wisdom, decided that I needed a few more challenges.

I was at the hospital one morning in June of 1992 and was cheerfully delivering mail on the second floor. I had just shared a joke with one of the nurses on duty and turned to hand the mail to Lorraine, the unit secretary. Something was suddenly wrong, but I couldn't identify what it was. I seemed to lose touch with everything and everybody. I had my hand extended and the mail fell onto the counter. I knew it was falling, but had no ability to stop it.

The next hazy recollection I have is of Sharon Kerner, a nurse on the unit who knew me well, holding me down in a wheelchair at the other end of the hall. She was loudly telling me not to try to get up. She was asking me other things, but I didn't understand what she wanted me to do. Though I struggled to say something, she held me down and let me know that she was in control.

The next thing I remember, I was lying in one of the hospital beds, and a familiar face, at the end of the bed, was looking down at me. She asked me if I knew who she was. I knew I did. But I couldn't think of her name. (It was Donna Levesque, one of my old nurses and good friend). After a few confused seconds, that seemed like hours, I figured out who she was. No sooner had I told her, than she asked me what her husband's name was. I was upset that she asked me another question so soon, without giving me enough time to think. I responded angrily and said, "How in Hell do I know what your husb..." then, his name popped into my head. I gradually felt really sorry, stupid and ashamed. Donna knew that I knew Tony very well and was in trouble if I couldn't remember his name. I felt embarrassed and humiliated.

I suddenly realized that Dr. Caldwell (the doctor who found me in the hardware store previously) was beside me and I had learned to read his face very clearly, much earlier in my recovery. He had always made his concern for my safety readily visible. I could tell that he was very concerned now. He had been the one who had always said "No" to me before. He was a gentle, caring, soft-spoken man, but he saw to it that I was restrained the last time I was "in these beds". He said "No", to my using the elevators alone, using the stairs alone, and traveling alone. He was the one who had said "No" to my flying alone and my driving, when I wanted to try.

Suddenly I felt fear sink into my stomach, as that possibility entered my head. I looked at him. I could read the concern in his eyes. I think he knew how scared I was...and I was not discussing anything anymore with anyone...end of discussion. I would rest for the afternoon and be fine by 4 o'clock. I left the room feeling totally exhausted and against everyone's better judgment.

About ten minutes later, Donna called me back and asked if she could hold the keys to my car. She reminded me that sometimes, I did things without thinking. Wasn't that true? "Yes", I agreed to that. She said she would rest easier if she didn't have to worry about my leaving in my car. I trusted Donna, so I gave her my keys. I didn't want to forget either, and drive in an unsafe condition. She promised that we would discuss things later after I felt better and she finished work.

Unknown to me, Donna put in a quick call to Gordon and arranged for me to stay overnight with her and Tony. It was not an unusual arrangement. Often when I was in the city late, and had to be back at the hospital early, I had stayed with them overnight.

By the time we left at 3:30, I was sure that I had fully recovered. But I left my car at the hospital for the night and rode home with Donna. I agreed that was probably a good idea. I had trusted her for a long time.

About 7 o'clock that evening, while I was working at her dining room table, I suddenly felt overwhelmingly tired. Donna was standing nearby, so I told her I thought I would go and sit in the recliner for a while and rest. She looked concerned and suggested that I probably should go to bed for the night. Even though it was early, it had been a long day for me. I agreed, without any discussion, and went to bed.

The next morning she told me that I had had another spell the night before. she said she had stood in front of me for several minutes and waved her arms and I only stared at the clock. When I finally came out of it, was when I apparently said I was tired. I don't remember anything happening at all. It is as though it never happened. Only the fact that I trust Donna so much, convinced me it did. We talked about the possibility of seizures occuring, and that I should see my neurologist. I told her not to worry, that I was fine. Besides, if I was having seizures, I would lose the right to drive, and I was not going to consider that possibility. She understood how I felt and just calmly said, "We'll talk about it more later, if that is O.K.?" I answered, "Sure, No problem."

That morning, during a physical therapy session, I was lying on a cot. My therapist was working on my shoulder and talking to me about a wedding. All of a sudden, she was talking about dogs. I thought to myself, "How did dogs get into our conversation about weddings?" But I didn't say anything out loud. Her face was ashen. She quickly got up and told me not to move.

I heard the call for Dr. Caldwell go out over the intercom. I thought to myself, "Oh NO! This isn't happening again. I won't let it...PERIOD!" Dr. Caldwell was out of the building, but Dr. Hull, another physiatrist, came in immediately. He looked at my eyes and said they were glazed. He told me that I had had a seizure. I said, "This is not going to stop my driving, is it?" He looked down and said "YES"...not "maybe", not "perhaps", not "we'll see", but "YES"! I was devastated. No one understood how much driving meant to me, especially not this doctor who barely knew me.

For the very first time in my recovery process,

I lost my desire, my motivation, my determination, and I felt as if I was left with nothing.

I started to cry. Dr. Hull left to contact Dr. Caldwell. One of my old therapists who knew how much I used music to calm me down, brought in a recorder with music and let me use her earphones. I turned up the volume and tried to drown out the past few minutes. My sobs wracked the room and I didn't even care.

I couldn't face not driving again. I decided not to listen to anyone anymore. No one in the whole world knew how vulnerable I was, when it came to losing the right to drive. I couldn't and wouldn't deal with that loss again.

Dr. Marks arrived moments later and talked to me. He explained that we would just have to meet this obstacle with the same determination that I had used to overcome my first setback. That was really easy for HIM to say. I never answered him. I coudn't stop crying. I was angry. He didn't understand either, that I no longer had the energy to go through it all again. Whatever magical motivation I had before was gone. My determination was gone. I didn't want to work anymore to get better, and then get shortchanged again. As far as I was concerned, it was over.

Dr. Caldwell called my acute care doctor at home a few hours later, and the decision was made by my team to send me immediately from the hospital to a neurologist for an EEG and tests. From the testing and observation, I was diagnosed with seizures and placed on medication. The neurologist said, however, that if they could get the medicine regulated, and I had no more seizures for six months, I could drive again in January of 1993.

I had calmed down by that time. I had even gotten over feeling sorry for myself. I had been able to think about the future with a little more of my usual optimism. Losing my license to drive was hard for me to deal with, but I still had a chance. After having gone for two years with only, "maybe's", at least now I knew what I had to do and how long I had to wait, before I could start again.

Everyone spent much time trying to make me understand how dangerous it would be on the road, driving if I had another seizure. I could understand that, but accepting it was altogether different. I just wanted to drive.

I went through problems getting regulated on the medicine. With my memory problems, often I would forget that I took it, and take it again, or I would forget to take it at all. I tried exceptionally hard to concentrate, because of my intense desire to return to driving. I was concerned that by the time I got back on the road, I would forget the strategies I had learned that allowed me to drive safely. That seemed to be the least of everyone's worries. Most believed I am sure that I was permanently off the road. I know many members of my family certainly hoped that was true. They feared for my safety, and maybe even theirs. But time would heal all the wounds.

The six months went by slowly. I looked forward to January 5. I circled the date on my calendar on the wall at home and starred the day in my memory book. Each morning I counted down the days to go. By January, Gordon, too, was hoping I would make it. The two roundtrips to Portland every Tuesday and Thursday were hard to get used to again, after driving myself for five months.

It was also gymnastics season once again and he was having to take me everywhere. I prayed every day that I would experience no more seizures or any other medical problem that might extend the date.

When the day finally arrived, he was more eager for me to return to driving than even I was. My wheels were under me and I could be independent again. As I put my car key into the ignition, I thanked God for being patient and understanding with me. I thanked myself for making it through the wait. I also said a prayer for Donna Levesque and Dr. Caldwell for keeping me safe. I was truly grateful and appreciative of their concern. I even kind of forgave Dr. Hull, who did nothing but be honest with me, at a time when I didn't want to hear honesty.

...And Dr. Marks, well, he always understood me. He knew that my tears dry up quickly and that my motivation was really indestructable.

*"Whenever a door shuts,
A window always opens."*

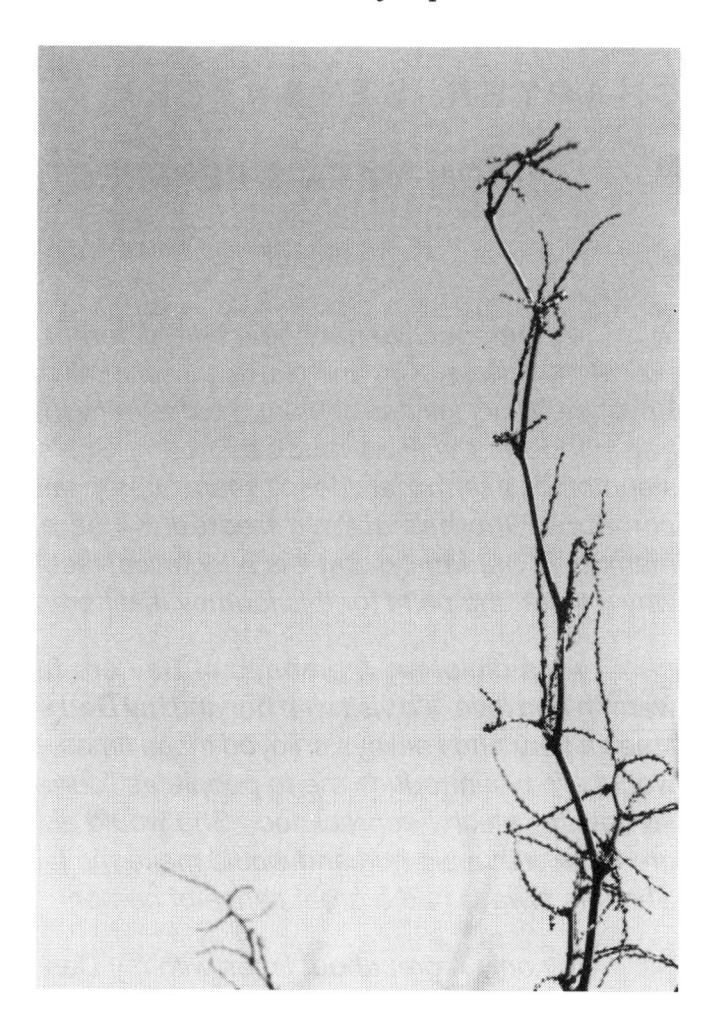

CHAPTER SEVENTEEN

FROM MARK'S PERSPECTIVE

My perspective may be a little different that that of my sisters, Kim and Carrie. First of all, I call Beverley, "Bev", instead of Mom. I've never lived with her, although I visit as much as I can. She's my stepmother, a term that doesn't seem appropriate for someone who has always treated me as a full member of her family. But it is a technical fact, and why my starting point for this journey is different.

As a child, my memories of Bev are full of warmth and love. I'd visit with her and my Dad a few times a year and I always enjoyed those times. Bev would always introduce me to people as "our son", something which I appreciated. She would always greet me with a big hug and would make me laugh. She has always had a great sense of humor.

My only regret about times with my Dad and

Bev, when I was a child is that there were not enough of them. That wasn't their fault. I didn't live nearby, and they did their best to see me whenever they could.

When I started at Northeastern University in Boston at age 18, the relationship I had with Bev, Dad, Kim and Carrie began to grow. I was on my own now. I had my own car and could visit whenever I wanted. And I did this often, doing things young college students do, like bringing home 8 weeks worth of dirty laundry. Bev would magically turn them into a suitcase of clean, folded clothes. During the 5 years I spent at Northeastern, I really got to know Dad and Bev like I never did before. We developed a bond which will not be weakened, even with my moving away from the New England area.

After graduating, I took a job with AT&T in Denver. There I met Hilary, who is now my wife. In 1988, I arranged a job transfer to England, where I currently live. This is where I was when I heard the news of Bev's accident.

When you hear bad news over the telephone, it can be difficult to make it sink in. My connection with Bev's first few months of recovery was a series of disjointed messages. The first news I heard was that she had an accident, but was basically okay. Then there was speculation about some sort of stroke. It was a long time (or so it seemed) before the words "brain injury" were spoken.

Each time I talked with Dad on the phone, the situation with Bev would be totally different. I would always ask the question, "How's Bev?" with the fear of what the answer would be. Sometimes, it was good news, for instance, she was now cleared to drive. Sometimes, it was bad news. She was no longer driving. Between the month or two that would go by between phone calls, I would assume that things would either stay the same, or slowly improve. I'd feel disappointed if this didn't happen.

When talking on the phone with Bev, she sounded so normal. The only thing that seemed different is she didn't want to talk for very long. But from 4000 miles away, Bev seemed the same.

I knew from talking with Dad that she was not the same. He didn't hide things from me and he did his best to try to explain what was happening. But this, too, was difficult over the telephone.

When I first traveled to Maine to visit the "new" Bev, I didn't know what to expect. Even with the detailed information Dad had given me, it was hard to visualize what she was really like. My initial reaction was the same as I had on the telephone. She was the same! I wondered what all the fuss was about.

She greeted me with the usual big hug, smile, asked how long the trip was, and offered me something to eat. Being a frequent traveler, Bev knew how unsatisfying airline meals were. But a few minutes later, she disappeared into the quiet of her computer room. Dad explained that the noise and excitement of our arrival was a lot of stimulation for Bev and she needed to leave to give her brain a rest.

Maybe things were not as normal as I thought. When Kim came to visit with her three energetic children, Bev would again disappear.

If I had to summarize how I see the "new" Bev, 90% of the time she seems the same to me as the "old" Bev. I'm sure I notice the differences much less than the rest of the family. The differences I do notice are the ones which are clear and frightening.

The most vivid memories I have of such differences came when Bev and Dad visited us in England. They had already visited us once before her accident and we had a great time showing them around the South of England and the city of Bath, where we live. One year after her accident, they visited us again and we toured Scotland together. Our journey started in Edinburgh, the capital of Scotland. We arrived in the city during the Jazz Festival and a day after the Military Tatoo. It was crowded. We went to Edinburgh Castle and left no 12th century stone unturned. It was upon leaving the castle that it happened.

On the busy "Royal Mile" street that runs from the castle, Bev suddenly bolted out into the road in front of a stream of speeding traffic. Dad ran after her and pulled her from the traffic. Hilary and I were shocked. "What on earth was she doing?", we wondered. Dad, of course, understood. While we were shocked with surprise, I suspect Dad was angry with himself for not watching Bev more closely.

He was obviously upset by the incident, but not surprised. This is when I realized that no matter how much Bev seemed the same, she was not.

We had a great time in Scotland, and there were no other memorable incidents, like the one in front of Edinburgh Castle.

These days, Bev is more careful in traffic. She doesn't run away to the computer room, not even when there are 16 relatives over for dinner.

The obvious signs of the "new" Bev are no longer there for me. Sure there are large PINK signs all over the house, helping Bev to remember various things. She sometimes forgets what we did yesterday. But rather than being 90% normal, she is now 98%.

It is far easier to cope with the changes, as they seem so minor these days. Because of the distance, it is far harder for me to truly understand what is happening, however, and how it affects the rest of the family every day. Ignorance is bliss, as they say.

I do understand enough to know that Bev has made an amazing journey and continues to do so. Reading IN SEARCH OF WINGS helped me a lot in understanding this journey. I have the greatest *respect and admiration for what she has done and is doing.*

I know the seas have been much rougher for my sisters, than they have been for me, but Dad, especially, made sure that the boat didn't capsize. While he can't change the course that the ocean may choose, he is constantly struggling to keep the family afloat.

ACCEPTING CHANGE

*Now is the time for believing
In who I might become,*

*And forgiving those who dwell
On who I used to be.*

*I cry, sometimes, alone at night
For what I might have been,*

*But then, I take the time to laugh
Giving thanks for who I am.*

CHAPTER EIGHTEEN

BUILDING LIFE RAFTS

GOAL THREE: My third goal in my revised vocational rehabilitation plan was to volunteer in many different jobs. I wanted to especially assist and work with other persons with brain injury.

When I was first injured I thought I was the only person who felt like I did. I went to a support group in my home area, but found that many people had different problems. Most had physcial handicaps that made it obvious to all that they had trouble functioning.

I had no visible signs that I might be challenged. I could talk intelligently and had a wide frame of knowledge and experiences on which to draw. What people didn't know was that within ten minutes of a conversation with me, the information relayed had disappeared into oblivion. No one saw that I couldn't function in crowds, because I had been taught to leave the room quickly. I used my schedule book to record everything and people often wondered why I wrote everything down. The hardest people to relate to were those in the group who had dealt with their injuries many years before, and were not familiar with the newer rehabilitation techniques. I felt I needed people who had problems like mine and understood the problems I had in dealing with issues.

One day while I was volunteering at the hospital, one of the speech therapists came up to me in the hall, and asked if I would be willing to meet with another outpatient and talk with her. When we met, we decided to form a support group for people who lived independently and were trying to work on their own after rehab. We organized a support group, called T.B. I. Voices. Our motto was "Silent no more". We decided that we would advocate for persons with brain injury so that they would no longer be relegated to back rooms or closets, or be afraid to speak out for fear of being rejected, or incompetent. We were proud of our new group and set about developing guidelines and goals to meet our own needs.

Being There

Sometimes I feel like that beachcomber after the storm, pausing every little while to pick up the pieces. Some are so broken, they may never be put back together. Some still lie unscathed in the sand, and look just as natural as before the storm.

There is a beauty in all things. Some sparkle in the sunlight. Others shine in the dark of night, while others have a special kind of inner glow to them. But finding one thing always leads to the hope and excitement that there will be another just ahead.

The driftwood reminds me that things survive, although sometimes, in a different form. I marvel at all of the other things on the beach after the storm. The rocks, all unique in their own way, many sizes, shapes and yet, none identical. Each one bearing the marks of pounding and rolling with the currents and the tides, becoming smoother in time as they tumble with the forces of nature..

We are all changing, even the rocks. Some because of the storm, and others, in spite of it.

There is a silent unity here, each left with changes, each with its own space on the beach, each with its own character, exciting, and sharing a sense of belonging to each other.

...

All are part of a greater scheme. United, we validate the storm, and in return, we validate each other and our own existence."

We wanted to be a part of improving things, and yet, still provide a forum for mourning our losses and sharing our feelings with each other. Although we started with two members, within a year our membership had grown to 17. We designed a logo and bought sweatshirts and tee-shirts with our logo and motto.

Our goal was to get the chance to make more people aware of brain injury. We organized a trip to Washington to see if we could take more responsibility on our own. We all came back exhausted, but we made it.

By 1994, over 93 survivors has passed through our group, and we had an active membership of 15-20 at every meeting. It was obvious that we were making an impact on the community. Members took part in a free skiing program for people with disabilities, while others went to conferences all over the country to bring back information on brain injury.

One of our members secured television coverage on several local stations and what started as a public information blurb grew into a full feature, prime time publicity for brain injury. We used the strengths of each member who was willing, to help us grow. Those who could write, wrote. Those who had artistic strengths, designed. Those who had computers, organized. Those who liked to read, read. Those who had time, volunteered in schools, churches, organizations and hospitals. We were asked to talk to other support groups to see if we could get them inspired, too.

Our members worked within the structure of the Maine Head Injury Foundation (Now renamed the Brain Injury Association of Maine), and served on its committees, and four of our members were elected to its Board of Directors. In 1994, I was elected President of the Foundation. It was an honor, and one that I knew, meant I had to eliminate some other things in my life. But serving and helping people with brain injury was a goal of mine, and it was all-important to me.

It was at T.B.I. Voices that I made friends; friends who replaced ones that I lost after my injury, and friendship between survivors is a very cherished thing. It is based on a common understanding that we have shared something unique that only we can truly understand. That makes our relationship intimate from the beginning.

JUST BE MY FRIEND

*When I climb out of bed each morn,
To start the day off with a smile,
I only ask to find a friend
Who'll talk with me a little while.*

*The world can be a lonely place
When friendships disappear. How strange!
Just a moment means so much,
To those of us whose lives have changed.*

*Time as taken much from me,
But I will make it to the end,
If you will only take some time
To talk with me and be my friend.*

    The support group grew faster than I ever dreamed it would. It actually grew faster than my ability to deal with co-facilitating it. I was running into problems with the large numbers of participants and personalities, and getting bogged down with the outward expression of feelings that emerged. I needed help. I would come out of meetings exhausted, panic-stricken or excited and all the other events of my day would be affected. If any confrontation or anger was involved, I would leave the meeting, shut the door behind me, and stand in the hall and try to recover myself where no one would see me.

I was a leader to them and leaders listen. They didn't know that I couldn't deal with conflict of any kind or two people trying to talk at the same time. I couldn't deal with loud voices or interruptions, like the intercom ringing, or late arrivals and early departures. Two of our members had met and married from the group. We had the usual problems of any support group including substance abuse issues, dating, transportation, and handling medical problems during meetings. Our members preferred to have no professional facilitators present. I felt responsible for maintaining a non-judgmental atmosphere, and incompetent in being able to.

So when I met Pam, my state vocational rehabilitation counselor. I told her that I needed some help with this problem. I was floundering.

She asked how the rest of my volunteering in different areas was going. I was working in the Pharmacy and doing copying for the administration. I had worked with the cash register in the cafeteria, and done some recording in the lab. I had done a lot of copywork for the therapies and finished folder projects for referrals and nursing.

I answered, "I really don't know. I don't think anyone would complain if I wasn't doing a good job, because they were getting it done for free." We decided I needed someone to supervise my volunteer work, evaluate what I was doing, and assist me in drawing together all aspects of my work experience. Pam recognized immediately that I needed support and provided help.

She approved a course in Support Group Facilitating at the University nearby, and I enrolled. I learned some ways and hints on dealing with some of the problems I was encountering.

She, also, approved KoKo Keller, a vocational rehabilitation counselor at New England Rehabilitation Hospital to work with me, in dealing with T.B.I. Voices conflicts and, also, to supervise my work experience on-site at the hospital. That was the most valuable decision that was ever made during my recovery, but it would still be a while longer before I realized just how valuable.

Within 6 months, our organization of meetings had improved. We had a formula for making agendas for each sessions by organizing a board meeting to meet an hour before each meeting. We elected a group of survivors who could help facilitate and made it a true group process.Together we developed a system to handle whatever problems occurred.

T.B.I. Voices began to take on a personality of its own. We became known as a group that DID things, shared feelings, educated others, empowered ourselves, and over time, we found ourselves becoming a family...a family that dealt with a diverse assortment of individuals, and therefore, a diverse assortment of feelings. Some people had traumatic brain injuries, some had brain tumors, some strokes, and some chemical poisoning. Some people were newly injured, while some were dealing with injuries sustained as long as 28 years ago.

Some couldn't walk, or walk straight. Some couldn't talk. Some couldn't hear. Some couldn't think or remember, but we worked together.

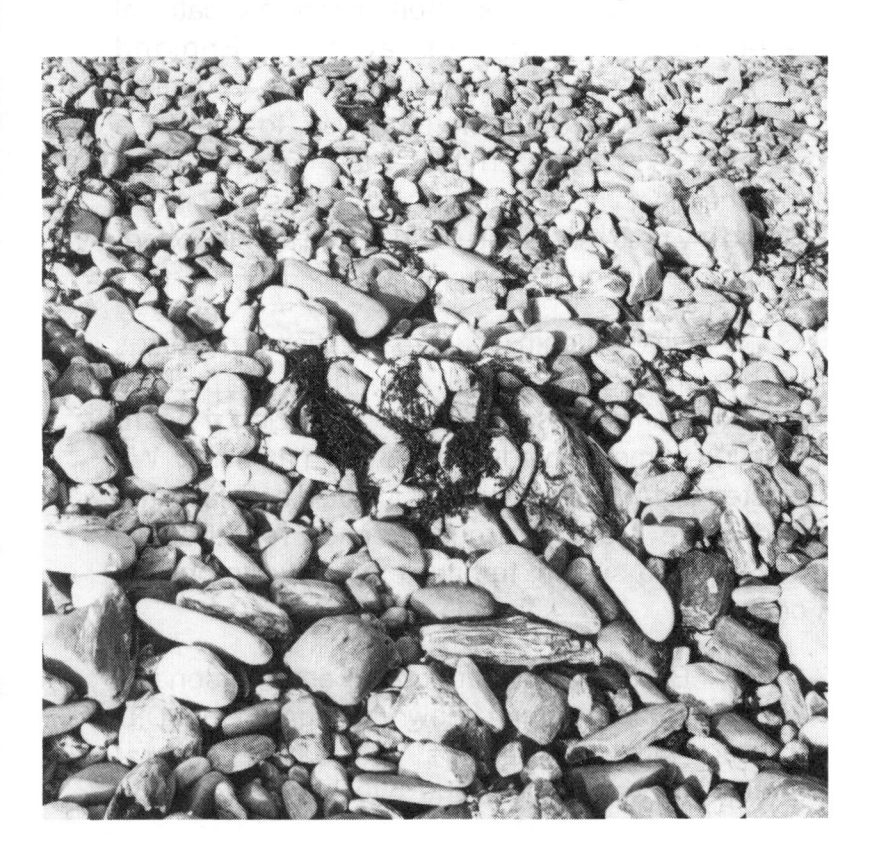

ATAXIA

There's a curve ahead

    that only I can see

        wandering side to side

    daring me to follow it.

If my trunk weaves,

    my feet fight to catch up

        Somehow part of me always

stays a little too long

    in one place.

APHASIA

*Sometimes when I talk with you,
It's harder than you see.
I try to find a single word
playing hide n' seek with me.*

*I know what it is, I want to say
And try so hard to sound.
But the word I want to come out,
Just simply can't be found.*

*I know it's somewhere in my brain.
It must feel so safe inside.
Because when I try to search for it,
The word decides to hide.*

*I know each word and all it means,
And what it's all about.
If only I knew where it was,
When it won't come out.*

Marcia is a person that I met in the group. She is an artistic and creative person who has been physically and mentally challenged by gasoline poisoning. She had late intervention, little validation and practically no help. She asked to write herself, rather than me about her. I am honored that she has entrusted her feelings to the permanency of my book.

"Bev is a friend I encountered on the crazy circuitous path of brain injury. We met when I attended a T.B.I. Voices meeting. My sanity was saved by the unspoken recognition of who we were and what we had become.

Since then, Bev and I have made angels in the sand together in the rain, floated endlessly in her swimming pool, while quietly acknowledging the world we have entered.

She and I have laughed at the deeds we have done, and held each other's hand in support of deeds we supposedly couldn't do. We traveled successfully from Maine to New York City, Washington, D.C., and Chicago, Illinois. We've spoken at Rehabilitation Hospitals, seen Broadway shows, and encouraged politicians to support brain injury funding. We understand each other's setbacks and are there for support, when either of us, or anyone else, needs it. That's what most friendships consist of, yet this one, is very special.

We are persons with a brain injury, yet we

are creative human beings, looking for pathways to express our uniqueness. We are intelligent people, hoping to be treated as such. It is all right to recognize that we sometimes have difficulty. Everyone does, with or without injury. We are merely trying to find our own way out.

Bev has thrown herself into the work of making life better for those with brain injury. Her level of intelligence and heart is greater than most healthy people I know. Nothing stops her and nothing ever will. She can make the world better and I feel fortunate to know Bev and to love her.

T.B.I. Voices has provided me with true comrades and a safe place to mourn my losses and explore my potential."
............................**Marcia Cooper**

I have met many wonderful, caring people through my work with the support group and talking with brain injury patients and their families. I have learned so much from the information I have gained,. and the professionals I have worked with. I have slowly relearned how to handle the situations that brain injury left me unable to cope with, growing so much in the process.

Part of the regrowth has been because of special people I have met like Marcia. Every once in a while, someone moves into your life and softly touches you. They do more to help you in the process of your "becoming", than you could ever thank them for. Such is the friendship I share with Marcia. She understands who I am and where I want to go. She walks with me and supports me. She worries about me and fights to clear the way for me. I plan to be there on that same road, clearing the way for her.

We are all changed. Everyone touched by brain injury is changed. Yet we all have something in common. Like I said,

> *"We are all driftwood,*
> *Left by a storm,*
> *That came and went*
> *With the tide,*
> *All of us, beautiful...*
> *Just as we are."*

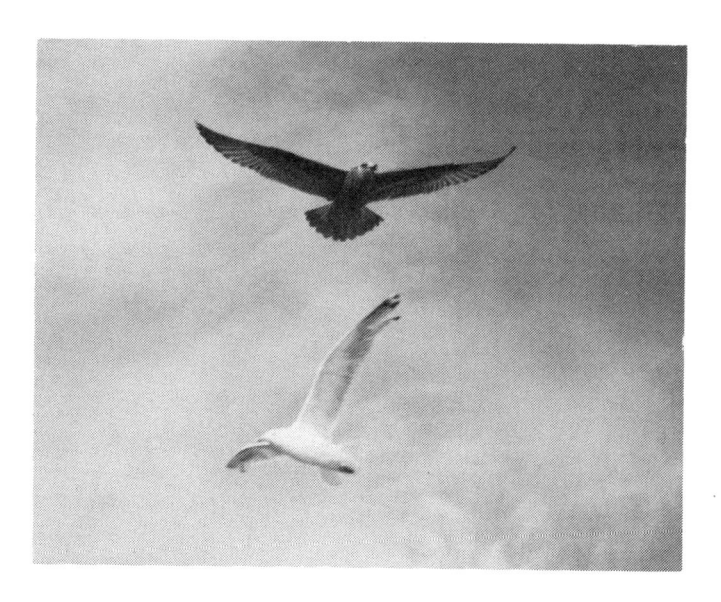

SECTION SIX

REBUILDING "ME"

SESSION SIX

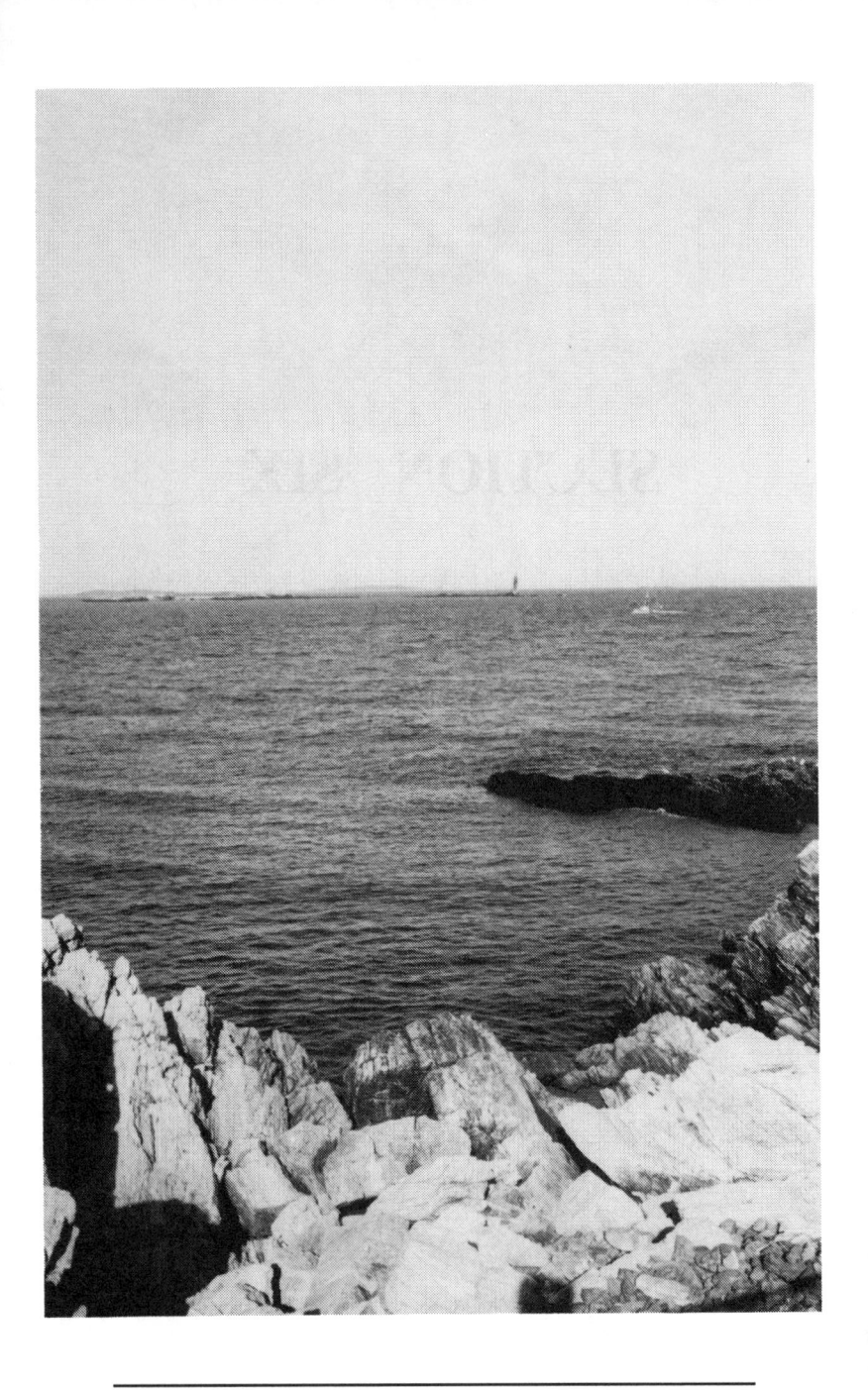

CHAPTER NINETEEN

RELEARNING TO SWIM

KoKo came to the hospital in the fall of 1992. She had no knowledge of my ever being there as a patient, only as a worker, and that felt good. One morning while I was doing some copy work, she came to the lobby to use the copier. As she looked puzzled, I offered to show her how to run it. Being a "born" actress, I'm now sure she already knew, but she gave me her undivided attention anyway. As I proudly showed her what had taken me so long to learn, the receptionist introduced me as a former patient and author. Suddenly I felt that I needed to prove myself.

That was how a woman, who was to have a tumultuous effect on my life entered it. She was vibrant and full of life. She reminded me of a cross between a gypsy and Auntie Mame...Both rolled into one body. When she was asked to step in, KoKo accepted my case as a challenge. At the time, I don't think she had the slightest idea just how much of a challenge I would be.

Very quickly, I learned that we had more in common than most people. My love of music had carried me through my recovery from brain injury and my enjoyment of music was a very important part of my life. KoKo sang professionally. I loved every single sliver of life and tried to enjoy it with gusto. So did she. I had choreographed many dance productions and she loved to dance. I loved the theatre and she was an accomplished actress. I was at my best when I was analyzing things. So was KoKo. We both were people who enjoyed making things happen, rather than just letting them. She was able to understand why and how I jumped into things head first. She did it, too.

She was an intense, quick-thinking, fast-talking task mistress. I knew from the beginning of our work together, that she would demand the very best I was able to give and would be satisfied with nothing less. She had a rare concern for all her clients and heard my cries and laughter with her heart, not only her ears. To me, that was all important. I could solve my own problems, if I could just learn to identify them when they were happening. Trusting her from the beginning of our work relationship, I knew that she would work to help me become more effective and efficient in dealing with other people.

I began to make progress with T.B.I. Voices. She worked with me to develop weekly agendas and solve the daily problems that emerged. We designed meetings that would utilize my strengths and make the job of facilitating easier. She helped us form a Board of Directors, worked with us on finding solutions, and she came to meetings to observe the problems first hand. She guided me through the process by taking the initiative when I couldn't or didn't. Eventually I would say to myself upon observing her, "Of course! That's what I should do (or say) in this situation. " It was like delayed insight.

She began to help facilitate at meetings so I could observe and model her. I knew what to do. I just couldn't recognize when I needed to apply what I knew.

In time, she patiently changed my tears into laughter and turned my moments of panic, that still happened often, into episodes of learning. She stepped into situations I couldn't handle and made them manageable. She showed me that I could still be effective in large groups, by staying organized, through pre-planning, and helped me with the mechanics of doing it, not just provide lip service.

We worked until late summer on finding strategies for making me better at reacting and dealing with crises, and gradually I realized that I, too, needed support. That was a hard thing for me to accept. I looked at myself as the leader I used to be, and failed many times, to realize I needed that same help I was offering to others. I needed pacing skills. I needed to be able to set limits. I needed reminders to continue using the strategies I had learned.

As I recovered and processed information at a faster pace, it was natural to become careless with strategies. When I was functioning fine, I wasn't aware that I was only able to do so, by using those strategies I had learned. So often, I would forget to write down things or not pay extra close attention to listen and focus on conversations. Then suddenly I would find myself lost and out of touch with what I was supposed to be doing. This was happening more and more, and I needed to go back to square zero and begin again. It is a very humbling experience, but one that survivors must continue to do if we are going to return to maximum levels of performance.

We constantly need to be aware of our own functioning level and set measurements for ourselves to evaluate how well we are doing. Otherwise, we cannot recognize our progress or lack of it.

I had problems making decisions. This was especially obvious when I had to order from a menu. Gordon and I dined out often on business.

I had worked on some strategies in speech therapy a couple of years before. I had been taught to make some decisions first. Did I want fish, pork, chicken or beef? Deciding ahead of time would limit what I had to deal with when I saw the choices on the menu. Another strategy was to select a restaurant that only had a few items to choose from.

Both of these strategies were difficult to implement in reality. Many times I had no input as to where I would eat, or after choosing a particular kind of entree or restaurant, I would forget entirely that I had made a choice. In fact, it had gotten to the point where I had resorted to ordering whatever the person before me ordered. I would wait for them to order first, and then say, "I'll have the same thing." It covered a multitude of problems and kept my inability to make decisions hidden.

That worked until one day my friend ordered liver and onions. I hate liver and onions. But I said, "I'll have the same thing." It wasn't until the dinner was served, that I realized I had to eat what I had ordered. I wish I could say that I stopped doing it. Less than a week later, the exact same thing happened again. It was after the second time that I swallowed part of that meal that I made a commitment to myself, to find a way to stop doing it.

So Koko and I ate often together in various restaurants, where we had to order from a wide variety on the menu. Some days we spent longer trying to decide what to eat, than we did eating it. But over the months, I improved. It was one thing to work on it in a therapy session. It was quite another, when you were actually doing it.

KoKo recognized my problems. She provided an atmosphere that was unhurried. We talked through many of the items, pros and cons, limiting the choices together. She actually helped me to deal with the process of deciding, rather than just the solution. Then after dinner, we would talk about the day, and she would try to stimulate my short term memory. She would share things with me about herself, and I would promise myself I would remember them. If they were important enough to share, then they were important enough for me to make a special attempt to remember.

I was determined that I would find a way to remember what she said. I knew that if I repeated facts and events to myself out loud enough times, I could recall them with a little better accuracy. So I worked on trying to improve my memory skills, by trying to remember everything she said. When I started for home in the car alone, I repeated over and over again what we had talked about. By the time I finished the hour drive home, I could still recall some of the information. I would forget it by morning, but at least I was working on it.

KoKo made sure that we talked about things I was interested in....facts, feelings, family, places, concerts, and people. We talked about Broadway shows, different kinds of music, our likes and dislikes, how I work with others and my business.

We talked about the value of change in my life, yet the difficulty I had in handling it. She explained how these types of changing situations occured often in the workplace and my need to recognize them before they became large problems. We worked on the importance of adhering to an appropriate schedule, taking into account my injury. She reminded me of the importance of being dependable and reliable, and not over-estimating my ability to perform. Yet, she never set limits on that ability and left me free to determine for myself, what I could do and not do, in the workplace or anywhere else.

She was a "people" person and her intensity kept me striving for more than I thought I could achieve. She was able to adapt her methods to me as I created new strategies to solve my own problems.

She respected my integrity and for that, I respected what she had to say. I listened and I modeled. She respected my ability during my recovery to set goals, and my determination to achieve them. I respected her for teaching me how to do it with joy and enthusiasm.

Since I had always been the teacher, I felt very inept after my accident, always having to be the student. I felt that everyone was teaching me, and I was unable to be of help to them. Learning had become a one-way process. She enjoyed listening to my perspective of brain injury and let me ramble on. She told me often that she was trying to better understand how I felt, thought, and perceived situations. I felt she truly believed that with her professional knowledge and my personal experience, we could unravel together some of the mysteries of brain injury.

She dealt with me as a friend, and I respected her as a friend as well. She challenged me on every front. I found myself questioning things I had taken for granted. I began to discover new ways to do old things. I had hated any kind of change since my accident. I wanted everything to be constant and consistent. I had problems dealing with things that changed. KoKo changed things on purpose. Then she stood back and watched me struggle to adapt. I thought I was struggling to survive. She knew I was struggling to grow. At times it was very hard knowing that she was watching me struggle, and that my deficits and weaknesses were out in the open for her to see. Then I realized that she was growing, too, by witnessing my struggle. By using original and different strategies, we learned together.

Knowing that I had problems with driving, she still allowed me to drive her around the city in traffic. She trusted me and I learned from that trust. She never told me what to do, but put the information to me as a question. If, for instance, I forgot to put on my seat belt, rather than remind me, she would ask me if I thought it would be a good idea if I put it on. That way I had to think about it and make a decision. Both of them, hard things for me to do. It, also, gave my brain a little more time to process and concentrate on an issue, increasing the odds that I might remember it longer.

Using the same strategy of questioning with my memory book, she would ask me if I should write certain things down, and I would decide for myself. Of course, the answer was always, "Yes". But, at least, I had to figure it out. She made it a conscious decision-making process.

She dealt with my inability to handle crowds and noise. I had not really had much experience with masses of people, so when surrounded, I silently retreated into my shell or ran in panic. The confusion and close movement was very hard for me to deal with. I still had a problem with my "filtering mechanism" when in crowds. I was unable to sort out the important things I needed to pay attention to from the unimportant. I suddenly became like a lost tourist in a strange country, trying to find the right direction in which to head. She purposely took me to those crowded places to see my reaction, and then we worked on solutions. We went to malls, stores, shows, the city, and conferences. We spent hours problem-solving solutions and trying new strategies.

We worked on many aspects of my deficits. I shared with her, things I would never share with anyone. She recognized times when I was drifting off and would immediately ask me what I was thinking. My answer would be of help to her in finding out what was distracting me, and of help to me in realizing it was happening.

Since I had been diagnosed with seizures and placed on medication, I had found it very hard to write creatively. I was taking 1200 mg of Tegretol daily and I felt it was affecting my thought processes. I told KoKo one day when we were alone that I was going to stop my medication, just long enough to work for a while on my book.

"Oh NO, you're not!", she replied. Before I could get my defenses up, she turned to me, and looked me right in the eyes. Grabbing my hand so I would stay focused on her, she said, "Beverley, How would you feel if I were in your car and you had an accident and I was killed?"

I felt the tears well up in my eyes and fall down my cheeks. My mind quickly visualized the drastic implications of why I must not stop my medication. I would be absolutely sure to NEVER consider that option again. She had, in her own effective way, seen to that. I was a very visual person.

She worked with me to devise strategies to allow me to work easier. We worked to develop built-in quiet times when I could think with less distractions. I utilized my music to assist me in relaxing, yet not drown out creative thoughts. She recognized, acknowledged and encouraged me to use my music, as a means to provide a more secure climate to get my mind into nurturing itself again.

We used music as a means of communication, of feeling what didn't need to be said. I used it to refresh myself when I was tired. I used different music to quiet my mind when I was over-stimulated externally or internally. I used music to help me come up with new ideas in my work and to keep old ideas in my head long enough to utilize them. Music was not only calming, but made me feel good about myself and those around me. It gave me strength to start each day and serenity to end each night. It gave me energy when I was drained and gave me a place to identify with when I needed it. Music was therapy...a great one for me. Koko recognized the importance of my music and we used it as a valuable medium to assist me in returning to the workplace. Is this really a tool to help people recover their working skills? What I have discovered is that whatever works for you, use it. Be aware of what influences you to be more attentive, motivated and responsive.

How many persons who have sustained brain injury need music in their lives? Perhaps all of us. Brain injury stops the music. Recovery involves finding that music again, in whatever form it takes. For me, without music, there is no song in the air and no spirit in my heart.

Each of us is capable of making our own kinds of music. Some use it to help them relax. Some use it to help them work. Some use music to dream new dreams or forget old ones. Some people never make or hear music at all. I feel sorry for those few. But for those who do hear it, there must be family, friends and professionals who understand and join in the singing and the dancing.

Music

*Music is the thing that makes me whole
It calms me and keeps me in control
Perhaps, I take a different stance
But music lets me sing and dance.
When I let loose, I take the chance,
That music is the mirror of my soul.*

*Music is that part I always share,
With ones I know who understand and care.
It doesn't matter what the kind,
I know it's just a state of mind,
But it's the only thing I find
To ease the rising panic that I bear.*

*Music is God's gift to those who know
That sounds and melodies don't always show.
Yet, if you listen, you may hear,
Variations soft, yet clear,
In tune, so they won't interfere
As other hearts once singing, start to grow.*

*Music is the flow through which life passes
Its joyous tones excite and soothe the masses.
Though we may be far apart,
If you listen with your heart,
I will hear the music start,
And we'll be joined as one, as Broadway passes.*

Music is my love, my life, my goal.
It calms me down when in another role.
Then lifts me up and keeps me where
The sounds of life are in the air,
Reminding me that I am there,
Within the music in the mirror of my soul.

It was KoKo who, also, recognized my dependency on George, my job coach in my original program, and who initiated the possibilities of changing my program to lead toward independence.

I was coming to work at the hospital discouraged, because I saw no hope of ever working my computer program alone. I had made much progress in just being able to get into the program and understand and utilize it, even if it was with George's help. He had done his part. I needed to move on, and nothing was happening, because I was not initiating any change.

Koko recognized my frustration and became the "shaker and the mover" who brought the team together immediately to correct things.

In the spring, I was a delegate at the International Brain Injury Forum in Oxford, England. I planned to market IN SEARCH OF WINGS there and had the book placed for sale in Blackwell's

Medical Bookstore during the conference. I did not go alone. I took my business partner with me to concentrate on the marketing of the book.

I received a lot of valuable feedback from professionals from many different countries, who purchased it there and sought me out to autograph their book. I was impressed and honored. Before we left I had the chance to hear many people (including Princess Anne) talk about brain injury at the conference. I had dinner at Blenheim Palace, and walked the ancient city of Oxford with a reverence of history unknown in our country. But the most challenging experience occurred on the way home.

While departing from Heathrow Airport, my carry-on was stolen. I laid it down for only a minute, but that was all it took. I lost all of my credit cards, money, jewelry and souvenirs. The metropolitan police wanted to know what was in my case. It took me a while of struggling to remember things. They didn't understand my memory loss issue. Later on the plane home, I went to write down what had happened and the security number of my claim. It was then I realized that my journal was also gone. It had the past three months of my life in it, and the schedule of the next three months to come. I came home a "basket case".

I thought I had recovered much of my memory loss. Once my journal was gone, so were most of the conference memories. But the most important issue was cognitively surviving the next few weeks. I tried other compensations and nothing worked. I lived in a state of frustration and confusion for over a week until another book was delivered.

KoKo put up with the panic and chaos that emerged and constantly came up with new strategies to use until my new book arrived. She helped me to put my schedule for the next three months together again.

My confidence slid once I realized my memory, that I thought had been restored, had only been achieved by compensating. It was another challenge that she and I had to deal with in order to get back to working independently.

She and Dr. Marks encouraged me to purchase a scanner that could be attached to my computer. Then each night I could scan my book and its contents would be saved. Just in case I should lose my book again. I wasted no time buying one and having it installed.

On the job, I found I was unable to work with certain kinds of noise. A radio playing soft music was okay, but a radio that was tuned to a "talking" program sent me into overload. I couldn't concentrate or pay attention. More than one voice in the background confused and irritated me. On the job it became terminal. If there was a great amount of movement in my immediate area or bright colors, I would lose everything and go into a "no funtion" mode or revert to an "escape" mode. An escape mode is when the only thing on my mind was getting out of there, and I usually did. We worked on studying when that happened and where it happened and then found strategies to cope or prevent it.

I worked on trying to be honest with whom I was working for, and telling them when I wasn't comprehending, so that I could work more effectively. I learned to recognize tasks I couldn't do, and ask for help. KoKo made me realize how valuable being able to recognize and evaluate these problems were, and how crucial it was to my successful work experience.

Because of my memory deficits, I had to do things differently. I needed to check and recheck my work hours and my assignments. Many of the things I forgot, I never knew I had forgotten and would have to be told. Then I would forget being told, if I didn't write them down.

Working with me was not easy, because I appeared to funtion fine, until you worked with me for a while. It was easy to forget my inabilities until I quickly reached a point where I approached incompetency...and sometimes, it was hard for many people, including me, to tell when I reached that point. To help me, you had to be with me in many functional settings and know what I was thinking and beat me to the problem. But once I learned to recognize the problem, I became very good at solutions.

It is very important that persons with brain injury are provided growth opportunities in the recovery process, beyond just a functional level. We must provide those ideas and challenges, as well as guide emotional redevelopment.

Emotions are the vibrators of creativity. We get creative when our emotions are in disarray. It might be loneliness, or sadness, or excitement that pushes that creative button. Up until this time, my creativity had been brought to the forefront, only by anger and frustration. That anger had produced my first book. Then, once vented, it left as quietly and quickly as it came.

I needed to write now, not out of anger anymore, but out of self-expression and desire. It was time I did it for ME, and not because someone else thought I couldn't. It was a time when I desperately needed someone to stir up that spontaniety to get the "juices" going, and kick the cobwebs out, so that I could begin to explore and create possibilities in my life. I had started my second book, TO WHEREVER OCEANS GO, but it had become rote and perfunctory, instead of expressive and dynamic. I needed that extra spark of excitement and enthusiasm to really self-explore my options.

By working together, KoKo helped me to understand myself and work out the conflicts and confusion. Everyone, with or without injury, has to deal with day-to-day living. But with memory impairments, and with concentration and attentional deficits after an injury, it is a very different problem.

She tried to prod my interest in self discovery, so that I could eventually solve my own problems. I had my own mind, my own determination and my own view on things. Her job was to mold that into a positive force that would allow me to concentrate my efforts on improving and creating new and exciting challenges for myself on the job. It was not enough that I just be helped to learn how to work again. I was retrieving my "old" self, who had been lost along the way. It wasn't a self that had been just hidden, and waiting for the rediscovery. It was a self that had been torn, shattered and annihilated after my accident, and had fought its way up again, from the ashes to a functional level. It was a good enough level for some, maybe, but not for me. I was not any better than anyone else, but I was very different. We worked together to help me better communicate my special needs to those who worked with me.

Hopefully those things we learned would help other survivors of brain injury yet to come, and other vocational rehabilitation counselors who would work with them. We worked hard on my work skills and at building a creative work environment that would challenge me. We did things differently, but the long hours that we exchanged information, shared ideas, and worked together helped both of us grow more aware of the complexities of brain injury, that we both dealt with daily in our lives.

Working with a team was very effective in

finding creative solutions, and KoKo was the link that kept that team together for me. She provided me with enough ideas to design my own work style, enough opportunities to try them out in the work place, and many times, just enough rope to hang myself. Then we'd both try to figure out why I couldn't breathe.

With her encouragement, I began to pick up and sort out some of the pieces of my life that needed work. I attacked life again on my own terms, and enjoyed the changes that were occurring in my job at the hospital. I became more capable of handling administrative problems in the weekly support group. The referrals from social workers, nurses and doctors for me to talk one-to-one with patients were handled with more dependability, confidence and understanding. I was learning to trust myself again. It was a very long process.

She worked with me on my schedule, so that I had more quality time. Better scheduling meant more free time. More free time meant less stress. Less stress made me more functional. It became a "life" cycle. It didn't solve all my problems, but it made more time for me to continue to write the second book.

No one, not even Gordon, had been able to convince me to limit ny gymnastics schedule, which had run rampant through the years and had become an overload on my already crammed schedule.

DAYBREAKS

*There are times when
I just need
To tune out the world
And rest.
So that I
Can attack it again
On my own terms.*

It had been the sport of artistic gymnastics that had motivated me from the very beginning of my recovery. Returning to the sport I loved kept me working day and night in the hospital. There was always a myriad of challenges to be conquered as the sport changed almost weekly. I regarded my return to judging as the ultimate victory over my brain injury. Even if to continue judging, I had to utilize many compensatory strategies, I cherished the achievement. I adored the sport, but not all of the time it took away from the rest of my life.

KoKo brought attention daily to the fact that since the marketing of my first book, I had many other things that needed my limited time. I could see the impact my book was having. It was touching so many people who had written to tell me how they needed help, and what comfort and education the book had been for them. She constantly reminded me that I really needed to put my priorities where they would do the most good for others, as well as myself.

Anyone could judge gymnastics if they put in enough time. But not everyone could write books that helped others. I needed to use the special gifts that made me different, to help those who needed it. Gymnastics had been good to me, but now I should make time for other important things in my life.

So I made the final decision to give up gymnastics. I am convinced that no one, except KoKo, could have ever accomplished that with me. My family had tried to convince me to stop judging for years, and many therapists had tried during my recovery before she came on the scene, but I refused to slow down. It was one of the hardest decisions of my life. I loved judging.

After 25 years of enjoying the fruits of my labor, I had made many friends around the country, and it gave me a freedom of being totally on my own. It was a passage of my life that I truly enjoyed. The sport, though it had consumed me, had brought me inner strength and self esteem. It was partly because of that satisfaction that I was now able to be challenged by new and other things yet to come.

I still miss it. I watch judges, coaches, and gymnasts I know on the television during championship meets and it tugs at my heartstrings.But then I thank God for the opportunity to have been involved for so many years in a sport I loved so much. It was a good passage.

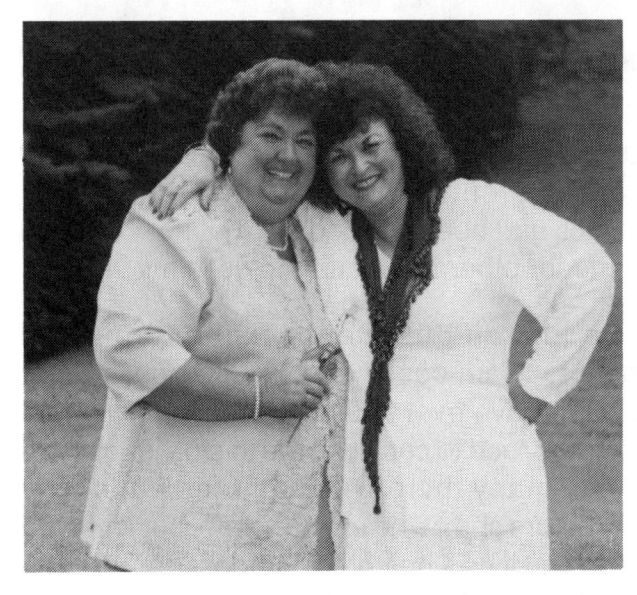

Bev and KoKo

When the requests started arriving for my first book on audio-cassette for those patients unable to read, I again turned to KoKo. She was a natural choice to be the reader. She understood the devastating effects of brain injury and she knew first hand, my attempts to deal with them. She understood the feelings and the anger that went into the book. She also understood the unquenchable motivation and spirit that continually carried me in and out of trouble throughout the book. I knew that my feelings were safe in her hands. I worked on my contracting skills and rented a recording studio and KoKo read IN SEARCH OF WINGS.

What an awesome experience to hear the book I had written, read aloud for the very first time. I cried as she read my words over the microphone. It was a true crying from the heart, almost as though the emotions were finally out. It felt safe, that someone who knew me so well and who I trusted so much, was able to "give "life" to those feelings. It was a very moving experience.

By this time I had developed a deep admiration for KoKo and what she had accomplished with me. I think she felt likewise. Working to satisfy the requirements of all my work jobs, I had little time for making new friends. I needed all the time I had just to get through each day. In working closely with me, KoKo became not just a team member, but my friend, as well.

I was intelligent enough to separate the professional and the personal times. For most people, this is not a recommended situation. For me, however, it was just what was needed.

I will not tell you that it was easy. We had to exert much energy to see that we did not allow our friendship to interfere with our professional work. There were times when I made mistakes in my work. I felt so badly myself about them that I knew she wanted to reach out, hug me, and wipe my tears as a friend, but she had to kick my ass as a client. She never hesitated to do that. She was a professional and above-board. Being first, and most important, a counselor with me, she worked hard to keep those times separate, productive, and goal-oriented. But then I was a different animal too. If my ass had to be kicked, I responded better to someone I trusted, kicking it.

One afternoon, after a very long and frustrating work day, I drove KoKo to one of the places where I often go, just to wind down. We went to the Portland Head Light, a lighthouse by the ocean in Cape Elizabeth. We didn't talk much. There was little to say. We took the time to smell the ocean flowers growing wild, there by the sea Silently we walked down the narrow, winding paths that ended at the rocks and the crashing surf.

When we returned, we each claimed a separate spot by ourselves. Lying in the grass, and overlooking the ocean, we listened silently to the sounds of the waves breaking below. We rested and we laughed for no reason. We even yelled wildly to the sea birds passing overhead. It was a release that comes only from nature and becoming one with it.

When we left, all the anxiety and problems of the day had dissipated and gone to wherever the ocean had carried them. We returned much more relaxed. Unknowingly, we had left our imprint there that day by the sea.

It was during times like those, I learned the most...about work re-entry, worries, emotions, friendships, about dreams and goals, reality, and life and how they are all interwoven.

I learned that laughing, with or without a reason, makes the whole world better. I learned that sometimes, it is not the complexity of what I learn but the simplicity that counts. I learned we must be sure to never lose those magical childhood dreams that make each of us so unique and special.

But, most of all, I learned that if I am to be happy and productive, I must take the time to reach up in excitement and try to grab all the stars. Yet just as important, I must, also, take the time to lie down and make angels in the snow and sand.

You see, the stars are for everyone. They are God's imprint he left for us to let us know there is a magic in the future, and our goals and dreams are there for the reaching. The angel in the snow is for me...a reminder that I am real and leave an imprint on the world.

In the summer now I lie alone on the beach, looking up in search of wings of seagulls flying past, spread out my arms as far as I can reach and make an imprint of an angel in the sand. It doesn't matter if the tide washes it away, only that I know how, take the time, exert the energy, and possess the desire to create it.

At other times, I lie in the meadows with the wild flowers and sing at the top of my lungs. Although I sing off-key and out of tune, it is only the wind that hears and hums along with me, as I leave my angel imprint in the flattened grass.

Some of my recovery has been an appreciation for that part of me that I leave behind as I continue to grow. The creative part of me was still lying dormant, almost three years after my injury. That "child" in me, who reached at night for the stars, and laughed in the day for no particular reason was, perhaps, the greatest motivator I had. That wonderful magical part of me that refused to see or accept the reality of failure: the part that dreamed of impossible things to do, and fearlessly tried to do them all.

The hopes and fervor of a child, still residing somewhere deep in my brain, were left innocent and untouched by my brain injury. For with brain injury we do, indeed, become a child again.

So it has been important for me to learn that at times, it is okay to be child-like and believe in my dreams. It is okay to be impatient and innocent. It is okay to cry and really need someone. It is okay to have a special friend and be one, too. It is okay to share the music in my heart and dance wildly to the rhythms of my soul. It is okay to be different from other people. It is okay to smile and laugh so that those around me do, too. It is ultimately okay to do all this, so I can work again in my own way, as I go and try again, to grow and fly again.

Even though I lost my creativity and part of myself with my injury, what is lost can always be rediscovered. Things are changed by self-discovery and I am changed. But now I am able to do it MY way, and to make things happen, so I can once again take control of my own life.

I am learning that I am a very unique and special person and have something of value to leave to the world. I may have needed to change how I did things during my recovery and apply different work standards. I may need to change things in the future, but I am capable. I may have needed help along the way, but I am learning.

It is my right to determine the work I do and the life I lead. It is my intention to share the laughter I have, the inspiration I feel, and the music I hear for those who are yet unable. It is my responsibility to record the pathway I will leave behind, for others to follow if they wish.

I think I have finally learned that life is a very special opportunity . My future is up to me now. It always was. So I reach for every star I see and lie down in the snow at the very first snowstorm. I know what I have to do, how to do it myself and love every minute of it. I can cry or I can laugh. Laughing is a lot more fun.

At sometime in our lives, we all need help from someone to remind us to remember to leave our angel imprint somewhere.

KoKo taught me this.

IMPRINTS

When time has passed, and I have gone
To wherever oceans go,
I only hope survivors find
My angel imprint in the snow.

One imprint made and left behind
Will melt and leave a larger sphere.
And if that's the only thing they find
At least they'll know that I was here.

But if by chance, they pass that spot,
And there is no imprint there.
T'was just I had no time to stop,
So I left it in the air.

CHAPTER TWENTY

REACHING THE SHORE

My formal vocational rehabilitation has been a long journey. It has been an exciting journey for me to be able to return to all aspects of my work.

What I have learned about brain injury and vocational services is that every recovery is different, because every person is different. There are no "canned" prescriptions or formulas for maximum recovery. There are no set charts to follow or textbooks that will apply to everyone.

There is no theoretical model for success. You cannot find the answers in a lecture or at a conference. Experience is, and always will be, the most effective teacher.

It takes many different professionals and non-professionals working with one individual to be effective. Successful rehabilitation is the art of building on each person's strengths, taking what works and utilizing it to the utmost and discarding what doesn't.

My experience is a real life example of what happened to one person, in one state, in one time frame. It is an example of how one team worked with one person, me. My rehabilitation program worked for me because of the initiative and creativity of those who were designated to implement it. They were able to instill in me a tremendous desire to succeed.

My first book, IN SEARCH OF WINGS, has been sold in all 50 states in the U.S. and is being read in 9 countries. It has been purchased by brain injury rehabilitation centers across the country for their professional staff, patients and families. I have received over 400 letters from people who have been "touched" by the book, and each letter I receive touches me in return. I have grown so much as a result.

In order for you to be reading this, my second book, TO WHEREVER OCEANS GO, must have become a reality. If so, it is a tribute that vocational rehabilition works. It is proof that there is worth in returning brain injury survivors to their potential. In doing our best to help even one, we at the same time are helping all survivors.

I know that vocational rehabilitation needs to supply certain things. One of the most important qualities is someone who really cares about the client; someone whom clients trust to follow through with plans and promises; someone with whom they feel free to share their concerns and needs, without fearing loss of services. Counselors must hear with their hearts and not just their ears. The counselor has to be able to effectively communicate with clients and be secure and knowledgable enough to recognize their client's uniqueness as a special individual. By working effectively together, much wasted time can be eliminated in returning that client to a productive work experience.

Physical skills have to be relearned and cognitive skills need to be re-established in order to be successful. Clients must realize the importance of understanding and dealing with emotions in returning to work, as they are determinants of success. Yet most emotional regrowth after brain injury is dealt with only when or after problems occur. Clients need to understand their feelings in relation to their work and their recovery, or they will not be successful or happy in any job.

We have to accept that vocational services not only include the worksite, but the ability to get to it (transportation issues), the conditions under which we reside (housing issues) along with many other issues that deal with our job performance. Are we late because we aren't dependable, or don't care, or because the bus schedule changed? Are we tired and need a break because we are lazy, or is it that our already impaired systems have become overloaded?

It is not a natural step in recovery from brain injury to become creative again. Creativity needs to be resown, fertilized, nurtured and cared for. For it dies a natural death, if uninspired. Those not so rare clients who are creative must be identified and challenged, so that their ideas become a part of the working solution. Otherwise those unfulfilled ideas will remain part of the problem. We all must use creative means in order to obtain functional outcomes that are meaningful, predictable and accountable.

For myself, I am extremely grateful for the help I received. Pam Williams was a wonderful counselor, in a field where compliments come hard. She fought for and defended my funding, understood my needs, and supported my goals. She firmly believed and taught me, that there are no such things as problems, only challenges. (She even asked me to write it in my memory book for posterity). Because she was willing to let me change and write my own goals, I had the motivation to succeed.

George Young, my first job coach, would have done anything to help me learn. He diligently helped me relearn basic computer skills that I had lost, and helped me understand the working of my business. He developed my list and check off systems that I could use, one step at a time. His constant smile and disposition were sources of encouragement to keep me plugging away when I felt like quitting. His willingness to go to courses with me was a motivation to look to other areas for help. When I couldn't figure out things on my own, he connected me with local resources.

My second job coach, for my more complicated needs, Scott Jacobson, made it possible for me to continue where George and I left off. He opened the door to total independence for me. His ability to utilize creative methods of training me, and writing a program that would utilize my strengths and eliminate my weaknesses were the marks that allowed me to move on independently. He was patient and experienced with physically and cognitively challenged clients. His many trips to my home and his insistence that I could do it on my own, helped me make my independence a reality.

Dr. David Marks, who was the reason I was able to return to driving, whether he truly believed I could or not, gave me the feeling that I could do anything, if I tried hard enough. Without his knowledge, his willing to test and give new input, and be a part of my team with Scott in developing my program, I would still be working with a job coach in my business.

KoKo Keller, my on-site rehabilitation counselor, still works with me today. She continues to restore my confidence by letting me see that the new person I have become after my injury is still changing, and guides me through the struggle and tears of the actual work experience on site. Her availability on the spur of the moment allows me the opportunity to watch and model effective techniques.

By encouraging the use of creative strategies, and her willingness to let me observe her own feelings, of anger, of frustration, of caring, of joy and sadness, she helps me to recognize, accept and communicate my own. She leads the team, finds the problems, and takes charge to see they are changed, while making sure that I stay on track and succeed. Because of her ability to adapt her methods of working to meet my specific needs, the creative cycle of self discovery is complete. I am a person I like today.

Working together, I think we learned many things in dealing with brain injury. What are some of them in retrospect?

We all have dreams and goals no matter who we are. Counselors have to be able to let clients know that they are real people, have the same dreams and goals, and deal with most of the same problems. They must be quick to recognize individual differences and set up programs to challenge all aspects of recovery, regardless of the nature of the injury. They need to work closely with clients in setting goals, assessing progress, and utilizing change. Counselors need to change as the client changes. Programs need to be revised, methods substituted, goals rewritten and procedures revamped. Success and change must become synonymus.

Persons with brain injury have to bring a desire from within themselves to be more than others envision and plan for them. We need to believe that we have the ability to do the job, yet accept failure as a stepping stone.

We must be willing, as clients, to be a productive member of our team and give our share of input and share our feelings.

Job coaches need to learn information first.

Then teach it to the client in a format where only the correct information is given. Persons with brain injury can not effectively learn by trial and error. All persons learn better in a friendly atmosphere with happy people.

Everyone involved needs to work as a team. If one part of the team breaks down, the whole team is diminished.

Last, but far from least, that productive vocational rehabilitation programs are like productive vocational rehabilitation clients. Each one is different. There are programs, counselors, and clients that will succeed and ones that won't. We must utilize what works and change what doesn't. I cannot stress that enough.

My vocational goals have changed totally, and I am excited, that my trek through recovery is helping others. I am looking forward to taking on even more challenges as they arise. This is just the beginning!

But I never allow myself to forget, even for a

moment, that the majority of persons who sustain traumatic brain injury cannot survive in the workplace, and never get over the obstacles that prevent them from finding meaningful work. We can't forget that most state vocational rehabilitation services have limited funding for many eligible clients.

Hopefully, insurance companies, the government and all providers will eventually understand, that people with jobs have self esteem and returning someone to the best they can be, is a worthwhile and financially productive investment in the future.

Persons with brain injury need financial help, medical care, services, validation and emotional support. All of us have a responsibility to see that they acquire that help, care and support.

Working as a team, we must make certain that future persons with brain injury, and unfortunately there will be many, will have role models to follow and leaders to challenge them. All of us, whether we are professionals, caregivers or have experienced a brain injury ourselves, need to do our best to see that we leave our imprint along the way.

SECTION SEVEN

THE WEATHER TODAY-

THE FORECAST TOMORROW

CHAPTER TWENTY-ONE

SURVIVAL TECHNIQUES

Staying afloat over the past few years has been an experiment in survival techniques. I've talked about the importance of strategies throughout the book. A strategy is just another way to do something, when the learned way does not work.

Some strategies I was taught to use by counselors, therapists and doctors during my recovery. Some strategies I developed myself in order to survive. In either case, they are survival techniques at work. Strategies allow me to deal productively with all the challenges I face. They help me to live day to day.

The ultimate goal of utilizing strategies with brain injury is to know when to apply them in a given situation and then, to be able to transfer them to other situations when the need arises. This is a very difficult concept to internalize.

strategies of communication

A few weeks ago I generalized a strategy and, better still, I recognized when it happened. Gordon and I have had to learn to communicate differently since my accident. Because we run our business from our home, often he would leave papers on the table after breakfast. When he came home for lunch, the papers would be gone. He would say, "Beverley, what did you do with the papers I left on the table this morning?" I would tell him that I had never touched them. In fact, I had never even seen them. He would get frustrated and I would get angry and defensive. Then later, I would find the papers where only I would have put them.

So we talked it over and decided to change our communication process. Now we do this. If he comes home and finds his paper gone, he says, "Beverley, if I were to have left papers on the table this morning, and by chance, you moved them, where would you be most apt to have put them?" Now, instead of being on the defensive, I have a challenge. I am encouraged to trust my instincts. I think for a moment, then say. "Probably on top of the fridge.." I go to the regrigerator, and BINGO! there they are. We are both winners.

Well, last week, after a day of changed plans and altered itineraries, I was driving North on the turnpike and getting ready to go through the tollgate at Gray-New Gloucester. I passed signs as I slowed that read "HAVE YOUR TOLL READY". I became frustrated that none of the signs told me how much the toll was. How was I supposed to have it ready, when I didn't even know how much to pay? As I approached the booth, I noticed that other drivers had tickets. My mind rapidly tried to decipher how they kept the receipts separated, from those who had tickets and from those who had none and paid cash. About that time, my car reached the tollbooth. I asked the toll taker how much I owed.

He said, "Lady, I need a ticket", as he waved a toll ticket beside my window. As though being a lady meant I didn't know what a toll ticket looked like, I said in the same tone of voice, "I didn't get one." He muttered loudly, "Everybody gets one". I replied in a louder mutter, "Well I didn't!" He very impatiently asked me where I got on. I repeated to myself, "Where I got on?" I thought...I couldn't even remember GETTING on.

As my anxiety rose 500 degrees, and I began to panic, I felt my foot going for the accelerator. I stopped and said out loud. "THINK, Beverley, think! Think! Think! If by magic, I had gotten a toll ticket, where would I have been most apt to have put it". Moving my knee, I looked down toward my ashtray. POOF! There it was. I handed it to the man, who was just shaking his head by then. I was smiling. He said, "That will be $1.80". I yelled "$1.80! Where did I get on?"

As I pulled away, it was an exciting moment for me. I finished my hurried trip with a contentment that only I could appreciate. I learned that my strategies worked and that I had finally internalized one, even recognizing when I had done it. So many of my frustrations and accomplishments have taken place at toll booths. When I need to rest, maybe that's why I love the ocean so much. There are no lanes, tolls, or toll takers to deal with.

strategies with panic attacks

I have learned to use survival techniques to help me cope with panic attacks, anxiety that has gone beserk somewhere along the way. The attacks started early in my out-patient rehab when I couldn't enter a room with people, listen to the sound of the hospital alarms, or people moaning at a certain level. My team worked with my re-entry into rooms, group dynamics, and eventually public speaking. That process took over a year before I was able to feel confident in my ability to use strategies that helped, and to handle social situations on my own.

Believing I could desensitize myself, I sat beside the alarms for a few hours. Soon after, the panic attacks began to spread to other things...the sounds of ambulances, fire trucks, police sirens, airport security alarms and transports, paging beepers, construction trucks backing up, and even eventually to my microwave, washing machine and dryer, and breadmaker beeps. After almost two years of trying to deal with the sounds, I was becoming totally dysfunctional. My panaic attacks were affecting my ability to travel alone.

One of my scariest attacks came in an airport while I was traveling with friends. We were laughing and talking together excitedly about our trip. As I started to pass through the security gate, the alarm went off. I don't remember what happened, but my friends said I took off like a rabbit. They retrieved my bags and found me later in an airport store. I was standing there wondering what I was doing and where I was.

After that, my secret was out. People learned how the alarms affected my work. My team worked on solutions, while I learned to recognize the problem and take precautions. Eventually I got to a point where I didn't worry about them. If I panicked, I would try to get away from the sound. As soon as I did, I was fine. I have learned strategies to cope with the situation. I know enough now to call home if I suddenly find myself in a strange place. If on busy streets when I hear alarms, I quickly enter the nearest store until they are gone. I have learned to ALWAYS keep my car stereo on whenever I am driving. Then if I hear or see a fire engine, ambulance, or police car with sirens going, I pull over and immediately close my windows. I quickly crank up the volume of my music until it masks the sound of the sirens.

I am now working with a psychiatrist who has diagnosed my condition as an "organic mood disorder". She monitors my medications. She thought my attacks might possibly be brought on by seizure activity and after talking with my neurologist, she started me on additional seizure medication, Klonopin. Once we reached a certain level, my panic attacks became milder and then practically stopped.

I still get excited at certain sounds, and get anxious during fire drills, but I am able to keep myself on site, under control and use my strategies.

My doctors have discussed other options, but in my case, apparently desensitization is not an option, nor is biofeedback. So I am relegated to long-term medication. It is a blessing not to have to worry about "disappearing" at the sound of a siren, or making a fool out of myself if an alarm goes off. Panicking is a very humiliating and terrifying experience.

I have made much progress in the last six months. I have every reason to believe that my problems are abating. By using strategies developed by my team, I feel I can travel alone now, with a sense of security that I will safely get where I am going. My team still worries about my traveling alone, but we worked it out jointly. I get to do what I want and they worry.

dealing with priorities

One of the most valuable survival techniques I have learned about setting priorities is there is a time to attack problems and a time to retreat. I need to know when to fight to change and when to reassess. Being able to do that can save a lot of time, energy and heartache.

An example of this happened a couple of years ago. I had not used my sewing machine since my injury, because shortly before my accident, I had lost the bobbin case. I now wanted to sew and knew I had to replace the missing part in order to do that. I knew exactly what the part looked like.

Gordon drove me to the store to buy it. The owner of the store said that my particular model, never had a bobbin case. I was sure that he was wrong. While he was talking, I noticed the part hanging in a package on the wall. I pointed out that it was the part I needed. The owner replied that I was mistaken. I argued vehemently that it was the correct part that went in my machine and insisted on purchasing it. I kept telling Gordon to trust me and buy it.

The store was 50 miles from home and I didn't want to have to come back to get it. He finally ushered me out of the store, while telling me that we would come back the next day if it was the part I needed.

Donna Levesque, my friend and nurse, was there and went home with us that night. After dinner, we brought down my machine and examined it closely. I wanted to show her that I knew what I needed. After all, I had used that machine for over

20 years in my crafts business, and I was ABSOLUTELY sure. Well, after an intense search, I realized there was no bobbin case on my machine.

Where the memory of that case that I remember to this day so vividly came from is still a mystery to me. But I allowed myself to cry, when I finally realized it wasn't there. Gordon tried to comfort me by saying, "It doesn't really matter anyway." Donna wrapped her arms around me as I "buried a bobbin somewhere in my memory". I cried hard, because I felt I couldn't trust myself anymore. If I felt so sure about this bobbin, what about other facts of my life, that I WASN'T so sure of. Maybe they were all figments of my imagination, too. That happens a lot with persons with brain injury. It's a wonder that we maintain any sense of confidence and integrity in our beliefs.

I told you this story because I'm now accepting that I can't always make things right anymore. But I have learned to retreat with my honor intact. Learning to step back and reassess is really a giant step forward. It is only when we learn to retreat, that we are able to fully reassemble our strengths for the next attack. The most necessary action toward success is being able to attack the challenges. Wisdom is gained as we learn to choose our own battlefields.

I have not used the sewing machine in the two years since that day, and may never use it again. Donna laughs about it now. I haven't got to that point yet, but that's okay, too. It's just another imprint left behind, or another challenge to attack in my own time, on my own terms, when I'm ready in the future. For now I deal with other challenges like scheduling, meeting commitments and pacing myself day to day. That is today's challenge.

dealing with memory

I have used strategies and made adjustments for my lack of memory. I use my family and friends for reminders and my memory book at all times. I use a tape recorder for important information and meetings, and I use no excuses for those times I forget. There are more important things in life than memory. Memory deals only with one portion of my life...the past. The past is always gone and I can't change that. I try to dwell on today and the future. I don't need all of my memory to do that. Sometimes it can be a problem.

I try to pay extra attention when crossing streets, but I still forget. Close calls have become a part of my life. But by using reminders and repetition, I am becoming better on my own.

I make lists openly, have pictures on my walls at home, utilize timers, and still use neon pink to get my attention. Wearing an apron reminds me to finish cooking and turn off the burners and oven. I am an expert on the use of repetition. I talk out loud and repeat everything I need to remember. I talk to myself over and over. It works for me and I am more apt to remember what I am doing or planning or where I am going.

dealing with driving

My driving has improved to the point where I don't have to worry about it anymore. For two years my car has been adapted to have my lights go on automatically whenever I turn on the ignition.. I have wondered if in time I would remember to turn them on, if they were not automatic. I found out the other day when I loaned my car to a friend for a few days. She turned off the over-ride switch for her own use and forgot to turn it back on. As I drove home that evening, darkness settled in. About 30 miles into my trip, I heard the sound of a police siren. I cranked up the volume of my stereo and pulled over!. As the policeman approached my car, he asked, "Ma'm, Do you know what time it is?" I looked at him and replied, "You stopped me to ask me what time it is?" He responded, "No Ma'm, I was hoping you'd turn on your lights."

My question had been suddenly answered. I explained, while staying perfectly calm, that my car had been adapted and what had apparently happened. I, also, showed him my brain injury card to validate what I was telling him. He smiled and helped me find the override button that would turn my lights on.

So I still have deficits that are probably permanent. But I can live with them, too. I've gotten used to the honking of the cars behind me, when the lights turn green and I don't go. I've learned to keep my gestures to myself when a driver cuts me off. I've learned to go by toll booths and make my turns from the correct lane. I have been retested by the motor vehicle department and they have given me the green light to drive.

It has taken me a long time and I've shed a lot of tears over it. But it's over. Gordon still has to remind me to do up my seat belt when I am a passenger. I do much better remembering to wear it when I am driving.

I still use a card in my visor to remind me where I am going. Sometimes, like people without injury, I forget. I still pass only one car at a time, and I'm very sensitive to cats. Perhaps, it is my guilty conscience.

dealing with "becoming"

I am excited about who I am becoming. I am more assertive and beginning to like myself again. Speaking in public no longer bothers me, and I feel very excited about talking about my recovery, my work, and my books. I am starting to take on my old personality of enjoying people and conversation and laughing. I am becoming a hugger again. It feels good.

Life is too short to not have a good time, and

enjoy every minute. Because of strategies, I can spend much of my time doing things I love. I have learned how to create again, whether it be speeches, artwork, crafts, music, or poetry. Sometimes it is fun to just create something out of nothing.

I still like to do things differently. I have espoused all along my recovery path that I was a unique animal. It is only in the latter part of my recovery that people are realizing how different. I now spend more time speaking at colleges, conferences, hospitals, and groups on brain injury from the survivor's perspective, and writing as healing from within. I like face-to-face relationships and the changes we have a chance to make.

Gordon and I are developing new interests and doing them together. We have tried hard to change how we communicate, so that we are both winners. We have learned what we say is not half as important as how we say it. We each do our own thing. He deals with the apartments and I deal with my bookkeeping and books. I wish sometimes that I could share more of the apartment work with him, because I know he gets lonesome, but I have learned to do the things that I can succeed at. At night our time together has become precious again.

Maybe our marriage is not the same as it was, but it is much more solid, and we cherish each other more. I respect what he does and he respects what I do. Because of my survival techniques, my family expects more from me and trusts me more to be independent and safe.

We cannot compare the past with the present, then and now. We have to live for today and plan for tomorrow. We are doing that.

As I learn more and process faster. I am trying to pace myself, say "No" more often, and take time just for me to rest. It works if I remember to do it. That is the hard part, perhaps the hardest of all. But setting my own course at my own speed helps. Once I do that, it is just a matter of "pulling up sails and heading downwind." I only need to watch out for the changing weather as time passes, and make allowances for it in the planning of my journey.

The process of "becoming" never ends. It involves everyone on the face of the earth. Strategies help us succeed along that journey, and allow us that precious feeling that we can make it. With help from many people, by trying different means, by traveling down various roads, we can achieve our goals and continue on our journey toward "becoming".

CHAPTER TWENTY-TWO

IN HONOR OF THE CREW

Persons with brain injury learn who their true friends are. I have lost some very close friends during my trek back. But I have gained many more than I have lost. Those who have disappeared had their own reasons for doing so. Maybe they weren't able to deal with me, couldn't accept my injury, didn't like who I'd become, or felt they had no part in my changed life. I probably will never know.

But there are so many things to do on my journey, and so many ports of call, that I can't take the time to feel sorry for myself or them. There's no need to. In some ways my brain injury has been a blessing. How many people without injury ever get the chance to recreate themselves? What an opportunity I have been given.

My interests have changed since my injury and some of my former colleagues have little in common with me now. We are going in different directions and at varying speeds.

My remaining friends have become closer and better understand me today. I cherish my new friends who are persons with brain injury, who I have been so fortunate to meet. They have become an important part of my life. We share something unique and special, that no one else, no matter how hard they try, can ever totally understand. Sometimes we follow each other. Sometimes we lead each other, but always hand in hand supporting each other. We have survived the storm together.

After injury sometimes, our old friends suddenly find themselves as part of a crew, standing on a strange deck. The boat has been refurbished, and the navigational aids altered. It is a struggle for them to stay on board.

Some of my old friends made the hard times easier. They not only stood with me in the boat throughout the storm, but joined arms in support, when the going got rough. Friends like Pat and Greg Zeitlin, who have been our close friends for over 27 years, and whose friendship I treasure. We have played over a million points of contract bridge. We have celebrated New Year's Eve together for every one of those years. We've ridden thousands of miles snowmobiling across mountain tops and trails in Northern New England. We have shared our family's celebrations of joy and moments of sadness over the years. They, too, have traveled my journey.

It is hard for them. I look the same, but I act differently.

Pat loves to talk politics, and I always take great pleasure in being the Devil's advocate. We have different views on many things and before my injury, I loved to debate options, and solutions. Not anymore! She is a perennial shopper, and I can no longer deal with crowds or decisions.

Pat is a very dear friend, who changes as I change, and makes adjustments as I recover. Her husband, Greg, continues to be Gordon's closest friend. Our relationship is even stronger now. For they have weathered the storm, too.

FROM GREGORY'S PERSPECTIVE

Before luxury

Before comfort

Before civility

Before living

Before existence

Is survival.

When I discovered that my friend, Beverley, was a "survivor", I felt frightened, angry and cheated. Her unspecified difficulties threatened a long, close and meaningful relationsip, we (my wife and I) had with Bev and her husband, Gordon.

As her problems unfolded and I began to perceive our situation, it became a burden. As Bev and Gordon changed, it became a kind of important adjustment. As Bev recovered, it became an exercise in living. As Bev began winning, it became a light of inspiration.

It has resulted in a different friendship. It has made us different people, somehow stronger, and maybe even a little better.

More than ever I am made aware of

The triumph of survival

The possibility of existence

The joy of living

The importance of civility

The pleasure of comfort

The luxury of friendship.

I, too, become a survivor.

..................Gregory....

Perhaps the hardest friendships to keep are the ones that are enmeshed with the work experience. The colleagues who develop a bond of respect in their working relationship and become friends. This was the core of my social friendships. I had many friends all over the state, region and country in gymnastics.

After my injury, some of them disappeared into the woodwork. My relationship became a perceived threat. Everyone knew that something was different about me after the injury. Because it wasn't something that you could see, or put your finger on easily, or instantly notice, some people did not know what to think. Some didn't or couldn't take the time to find out. Some were truly worried about being alone with me in a car, miles from anywhere, in case of a medical emergency or not knowing what weird behavior I might exhibit. I felt myself slowly losing their trust in my judging ability, even though I was totally honest with them.

Sometimes I felt maybe too honest. I have now learned to discuss my injury at times, and not to discuss it at other times. Sometimes it is better to say nothing.

Martha Butler, called "Marty", has been a very long-standing friend of mine for many years. We have been through a lot together. Our friendship survives despite the change in me, but Marty has to, also, deal with the memory of the person I used to be.

FROM MARTHA'S PERSPECTIVE

My name is Martha Butler. I am a friend and gymnastics colleague of Bev's. My daughter was a gymnast and I wanted to learn more about gymnastics and the scoring procedure. I attended a clinic that was conducted by Bev, who was the the State Judging Director. That was 14 years ago and just the begining.

During most of those years, Bev was grooming me for her position. We traveled throughout the United States to clinics and symposiums and meets. Part of our trips were to learn the new rules and to introduce me to the people with whom I would be working. But the best part of our trips were the spontaneous and crazy things we would do. It seemed that life couldn't get any better. Upon our return, the rest of our colleagues and friends could not wait to hear about the wacky things we did. More than once, it was said that Bev should write a book about our experiences.

When Bev suffered her injury, my first concern was of physically losing my friend. Once she was on her way to recovery, I then began to wonder if our life would ever be the same.

Shortly after her injury, Maine was going to host the National Judging Symposium in conjunction with New Hampshire. We had made a commitment before her injury and the thought of canceling was never an option. Coordinating such a massive event is a major undertaking for anyone. Bev dove into it head first, taking the responsibility for almost everything, single-handed. Other officials wanted to help and she was becoming exhausted.

In the past, we had an open and honest relationship. We could agree to disagree, say pretty much what was on our mind to each other, and then move on. I could have said, "Look, you can't do it all yourself. Let some of the others help." She probably would have mumbled and sputtered, and then said, "Okay, they can do this or that."

But during this time, if someone at the hospital, a well-meaning friend or relative, would point out that she was no longer capable of doing a certain task, she would become frustrated, begin to cry, and express some self-doubt.

This was to be the hardest time I would go through. We were right in the middle of the symposium planning and I realized Bev was no longer the person I was used to dealing with. I did not want to contribute to her pain, but I could not let things get out of control. I didn't know where to go or what to do. If I told the hospital staff, who were already trying to make her slow down or quit, it would only make matters worse.

I had already been called in several times by her therapists to be told that Bev could not do certain things, and that I should know better. Then Bev would tell me that she knew what she was capable of doing and not to listen to them. Since I knew her, better than I knew them, and I knew nothing about acquired brain injury, I believed Bev.

I didn't want to burden her family, because I knew they were already concerned enough about her, being over-protective at times. I was afraid it would only make everyone feel even worse.

If I said something to the symposium committee, would I be betraying my friend? How much should they know, and is it my business to tell them? I wanted Bev to tell me what to do, but I knew that was not going to happen, so I had to make my own decisions.

I decided to work quietly behind the scenes, keeping everything as low-keyed as possible. If there was a problem, we would steer Bev in the other direction and then deal with it. When some committee members realized that things were not quite the way they expected, I took some heat. I told them as long as they directed their anger at me, Bev was quite capable of running the symposium. If you shouted at Bev, she would run away. After all the work and preparations, I couldn't have them do that to her. There were a couple of close calls, and one day we even ran away together to buy a blouse.

It was a successful week. Bev achieved her goal in making it the best symposium ever. It might seem like the perfect ending, but now I realized there was another problem. Conversations with Bev turned to , "I did this" or "I was able to pull this off". But she hadn't done it alone as she thought.

I was beginning to wonder if there would ever be an end to the feeling that I must hide things or protect her from knowing the truth. I was also beginning to wonder if it was because she was unable to deal with it, or if it was because I couldn't deal with telling her. Am I being fair to her by not being honest? What happened to the relationship we had? Now I was beginning to feel like I had to analyze every comment to determine what reaction it might cause.

After the symposium I was emotionally exhausted, and I cried for several days. It was summer, and we would have a break for a couple of months. I needed this time to recoup. I had kept saying to myself that Bev would be the same person she was before. I even convinced myself, it was possible. I was just beginning to realize that there would be improvements in her condition, but she would never totally be the same as before. I missed my friend.

Bev was improving and wrote the book that our colleagues recommmended she write so often. It was not about our gymnastics adventures, although she did mention some of them in it. Her book was about the road to her recovery from brain injury.

This opened a new chapter in our relationship. We became partners and set off on this new road together. I now attended different kinds of clinics and symposiums. On occasion, speaking about our relationship, attending the sessions and learning how much professionals do and do not know about acquired brain injury. We were involved in marketing and selling her book, traveling once again...Boston, Chicago, Washington, England...........

Bev has become a very well respected communicator for persons with acquired brain injury. She has often stated that when she wrote her book, she had no idea of the impact it would have on survivors, families, friends, and professionals. This has given her a real sense of purpose and she can see the tremendous good, her work is doing.

However, with us, things are still different. When we travel, there are less, if any, of those wild and wacky stories. She would either be speaking at a session, or attending a session, and I would be selling the book, or attending a different session. We would see very little of each other. By the end of the day, she would be exhausted, and sometimes, fall asleep in mid-sentence.

In the past, when we were judging gymnastics, we both shared a dream. Communicating about acquired brain injury is a passion that is near and dear to Bev's heart. I was feeling guilty, because I did not share the same passion. When I attended the functions, the excitement is there, because Bev is what is near and dear to my heart, and she knows that I will do anything she needs or wants to support her.

It has taken me several years to tell her how I feel. We have both changed since her injury. The one thing that has not changed, is our friendship. It was built on a foundation of trust and respect for each other, and no matter what happens to us, physically or mentally, it will always be there.

I now realize that although we may be traveling along this new road together, there will be times when we will venture down different pathways. We both have different goals and dreams now, and that's okay.

There is no way of knowing if this is just part of a growing process, that would have occured regardless, or grew from the changes after Bev's injury.

Bev and I may not work or play together the same as before, and we may never do that again. But one thing I know is that I will never lose my friend.

.............MARTY..............

Making friends after brain injury is hard enough, but keeping old ones is just as difficult. People who are not trained in brain injury have an especially difficult time trying to adjust.

I also cherish the health professionals who I spent so much time working with and who left within me, a part of them. There is something that bonds people to closeness. It thrives only in people who have a heart with ears, who have the empathy to understand, and give the extra time needed to be a "special" person. Sometimes, it begins with the dependency of one on the other. But, if so, it leads to a stronger independence for both. Donna has been a special person to me since my initial injury.

FROM DONNA'S PERSPECTIVE

I'm sure that it is not necessary to preface this by saying I am not a writer. It will become apparent very quickly. What I am is a registered nurse and a friend. I have been a nurse since 1965, so I have worked with many patients. I work on the second floor unit of New England Rehabilitation Hospital.

Three days prior to my nursing school graduation, I was involved in a one vehicle accident, resulting in a broken nose, broken neck and a closed head injury. During this time I met the man I later married. He took the x-rays that diagnosed my broken neck. I'm telling you this so you can understand why I bonded with Beverley so easily.

When I first met her, I was her nurse. She was a patient brought to the TBI Unit of the hospital, because of a brain injury she had sustained. When Bev was admitted, it became apparent very quickly that she wanted her independence. Not that everyone doesn't, but even through her confusion and memory problems, she worked so diligently, that it became obvious to everyone that she would somehow, eventually succeed and overcome her deficits. Whenever roadblocks appeared in her recovery path, she rolled over them with humor and determination. Her frustration and hurt were worked through, and over and over again she persevered.

I can't begin to describe her feelings as she was the one who lived them. What I can describe is my admiration for her. I knew from the beginning of our relationship that Bev was a very unique individual and a very special person.

The day she was admitted, she told me about a trip to New Zealand and Australia that she and her husband had just taken prior to her accident. I really thought that she was fabricating, until the pictures were brought in. I was in awe. She told me about the job she had as a gymnastics judge, and the amount of frequent flyer miles she had accumulated in traveling for gymnastics. It was hard to believe anyone could have traveled that much. She had!

Bev was confined to a wheelchair, but she wanted for so long and so badly to get up and try to walk. One Sunday afternoon, when it was quiet, the staff finally gave in. We positioned her wheelchair by the nursing station desk, and I assisted Bev to her feet. She held on to the desk, and I stood behind her. At the time, her right leg was not strong and she had poor control in "swinging it through" to walk. I used my right foot to advance hers. She thought she was doing all of it herself. We walked the length of the counter. This was such an uplift for her, that we all felt the pride when she said that she knew all along that she could do it.

Bev made all of her achievements such a joy to all who cared for her, even though some of her progress made our job more of a challenge.

She never accepted things as they appeared. She always asked why or figured things out for herself. The biggest challenge for everyone came when she figured out that tinfoil blocked the alarm system. She really kept us running. We laugh often even today when thinking about them all. I remember how she disappeared into her cassette headset, when problems became too much. We shed tears together and a large hug at her eventual discharge. Her parting gift, a huge wastebasket lined with tinfoil, containing fruit, individually wrapped in tinfoil and hershey kisses was very appropriate.

A few months later, my husband Tony and I accompanied Bev and Gordon on a trip to New York. At that time, I was still in transition with my role with Bev. She was my dear friend, but at the same time, I was her nurse. What part of me went to New York? A lot of both. The "friend" part of me completely enjoyed her company and graciousness in showing me New York. The nurse in me died each time she was too impulsive crossing streets or boarding the subway. The bottom line is that she handled all obstacles and when I could become the objective observer, I realized that everyone else on New York streets and subways must have had the same brain injury as Bev. They too, were all impulsive and crossed between lights and were lost in their own world.

About a year after her inpatient discharge, and while she was still in outpatient therapy, she was visiting my home for a day. She was sitting on my living room sofa and, in a very rare mood for Bev, she was not her jovial self. I asked her if she wanted to talk about whatever was bothering her. She slowly opened up and told me how she didn't like who she had become...how she used to be able to do things so fast, and think so differently, do so many things at once, and have a "handle" on everything at the same time. Nothing ever fazed her. She was confident, dependable, and she liked who she was. But now, she said, she felt like she was a different person, and she didn't like the person she had become. I could tell she was very serious and really believed what she was saying. I also knew that this was a very hard thing for her to reveal to even me.

I looked her in the eyes and told her, that I never knew the person she was describing. I only knew this new person that she was now. THAT was the person I had come to admire and love as a friend. I asked her if she thought I was such a bad judge of character? She looked over at me and was silent for a minute. I could hear the wheels clicking. "Donna", she said, "You know, I never looked at it that way. I really trust your judgment; therefore, I guess, I can't be so bad", and she apologized. I knew that I had made her think.

Bev mentioned her old self, many times after that day, but never in the same context again. It was always for explanation or to add humor to a situation.

I've known Bev for five years, and I wouldn't trade her friendship for anything. She trusts me and my judgment, which is something I hope I can always live up to. I plan to be there for her whenever she needs me. The relationship now is not as patient/ nurse.

Bev, Gordon, Tony and I went to Hawaii together a few months ago. We spent 13 days on four islands. I realized how much things have changed. Bev, being the frequent flyer, was supporting me now, as I hate to fly.

We enjoyed the beauty of Polynesian landscapes, flowers and wildlife. We shared the constant sunshine and breath-taking rainbows. We watched the sun rise over the surf and set through the silhouetted palm trees. We enjoyed our vacation as friends, a friendship that makes me richer as time passes.

Between the laughter and adventures, Bev

made sure we left imprints on each beach we visited. I wondered at first, why she insisted we take the time to lie down in the black sand and white sand, and even in the rain, leaving angel imprints on the shore...imprints of a friendship, made from pebbles of sand, and coming from the heart. When I asked her, she just smiled and said "Let's just do it."

That angel in the sand was very important to Bev. It probably was washed away with the next tide, but that made no difference to her. As a result, what we brought home was even more special. An imprint of friendship that will last, that is nurtured by respect for each other, preserved by caring for each other, and that nothing can wash away.

...Donna

Today I am friends with many of my former therapists. We all have different relationships. They have been a special strength and memory that I have drawn from when I needed to. I have a much greater understanding and appreciation of professionals and know how much they, themselves, are affected by the brain injury community they serve.

Few people will ever develop friendships with the professionals who treat them, but everyone can work in a therapeutic relationship that is friendly and caring.

I am also making new friends on my own. Marcia Cooper, who I met at the support group remains one of my dearest and most precious friends today. She and I navigate together as we continue to peruse and pursue an education through brain injury.

Those who know I have changed, but didn't know me before, accept me as they perceive me today. They can make no comparisons to who I used to be. They are the hardest friends to make, because they start from that square zero I talked about before, and make relationships that give us worth. They are the ones who allow me to believe in myself. They have no pre-set expectations for me to live up to. They meet me and we go on from there.

I never expected to meet Ann Cox as a friend.

FROM ANN'S PERSPECTIVE

A New Friend

Bev and I hang suspended by our arms from the edge of the pool. "Poaching", she calls it. She tells me stories of her life. How she raised her children. How she and Gordon balance each other in their different styles, and while she talks, I hear his respect for her, her respect for him, their mutuality, and the wide freedom they give each other to be who they are. I hear how Gordon has stayed beside her, adapting to her changed ways without taking from her, that respect they started with. I hear how hard the struggle has been for her to reconnect with that essential self-respect as she comes to grips with her changed self. I hear of her adventures and escapades. How she dove under layers of ice just after recovering from pneumonia. How she traveled every weekend to judge gymnastics. How her interest in her students, her curiosity about the way bodies move through space, about the dynamics of gymnastics, and her ability to identify with precision each minute moment of the movement sequence, led her to become an elite national gymnastics judge. We share views on child-rearing, on spirituality and religion, on taking chances, on careers, and on life stage transitions.

I came to the realization as we talked, and said it right out loud. "You are one of the healthiest people I know." She was, I think, shocked by my simple statement and deeply touched. In her response to the statement, I began to realize the context in which she heard it. Since her accident four years ago, she had been in and out of the hospital, almost continuously receiving some form of medical treatment or the other. She had been grappling with physical losses, but most of all, dealing with her cognitive processing.

In the quiet moments that followed, I thought, our culture, rooted in European philosophy, doesn't often question the assumption, "I think, therefore I am." But what happens when the thinking part of person suffers damage? Do we turn the sentence around and believe, "I can't think, therefore I am not?"

So what happened to Bev, a competent,

mature person with well-developed self esteem, full respectful relationships, and an exceptional ability to see clearly and communicate compassionately, when the thinking part of her was injured? I asked, "Bev, what happens to a person's self image when they have a brain injury?" The response came back in a single word spoken with great intensity, "Shattered".

Bev's ability to think prior to her accident was something she and the rest of the world took for granted. Blessed with superior intelligence, Bev said, "I always waited for others to catch up to my thinking. Now they have to wait for me."

I reviewed what I knew of Bev before this trip to Florida. I knew little about brain injury rehabilitation, and because Bev was not "my patient", I did not seek to get to know her. I barely remember her stay in the hospital. I vaguely remember that she seemed very much a "patient" in that passive recipient of medical expertise sense of the word.

I do not necessarily believe that this is how other professionals saw her, but I am sorry to admit that I was content to role-label her and made no effort to go beyond this.

Sometime after transition from inpatient care to outpatient status, I encountered her at the copier, as she carried out her volunteer activities. She would always defer to my more urgent needs and step aside from her own tasks to allow me to rush through. Her eyes were very expressive, but I hardly stopped to notice, except in retrospect. They communicated both uncertainty and a serious determination. Sometimes she would smile shyly, but I had no clue what wit and humor lie beneath the surface.

In November of 1993, I was to attend a conference in Orlando. As I prepared to go, someone mentioned that Bev was to attend a brain injury conference starting the day mine ended, at the same hotel. Since I was going alone to my conference, I looked forward to having company during the evening hours and made plans to meet her there.

After a long day of presentations on chronic pain, I returned to my room and called Bev and her colleague. "Where do you want to go?", she asked. I had never been to Orlando and they had been many times, so we decided that they would show me Disney World. What an adventure this turned out to be! Thunder Mountain! It's A Small World! Main Street! The parade! We crammed as much as we could in.

Although I had moments of thinking that I, as a nurse, should be taking care of them as patients, I am happy to report that those moments were very brief. We laughed and played. One moment we would rehearse out loud what time and where we would meet the bus. (cognitive coping strategies) The next moment we would be talking about intellectual understandings about the meaning of life or sharing insights about human nature or tidbits from our personal lives as we became acquainted.

On the bus on the way back to the hotel, Bev beamed at us and said, "So who's going swimming with me?" "When?", I asked. "Right now. I'll meet you in the lobby on the first floor in 20 minutes." Her colleague began to protest about it being late, and I commented that it had been a long day and I had to get up early. "Well, I'm going anyway", Bev said. "You're the ones who will miss out."

Well, that was as close to a dare as it needed to be for me to change my mind and decide to go for the midnight adventure. What a great feeling to be under stars on a balmy night in a pool. What a gift! Well worth the effort.

That was the beginning. For the remainder of the time, I attended the formal conference in the daytime and spent the evenings, learning by experiencing. I learned the difference between thinking and being. I imagine that everybody who has had a brain injury, also, has a hard time sorting out the difference between thinking and being. I imagine that all their friends and relatives do, too.

Bev is such an incredible source of inspiration to others who experience a brain injury, professionals, and friends and family alike, because, with great desire, she has come to a new and fuller understanding of herself in relation to her thought processes. She has been able to gradually reconnect with and expand her own sense of self and self-esteem.

It has taken great effort, wonderful support, and good rehabilitation. But most of all, it has taken Bev's incredible determination and zest for life. She has always responded with energy, enthusiasm and insight to life, and continues to do so. For Bev, it seems, every day is special and my experience of being around her, is that spending time with her, makes my day special, too.

She said to me once. "I have friends who knew me before my brain injury. They see the changes and take my new state into consideration. I have friends in the course of working together on my rehabilitation. You are the first friend to be made with my new self" I am honored that she calls me her friend, and my life is enriched by her friendship.

........ANN........

I know I am more secure with myself now.

Part of it is because of many of the people who worked with me. Sue Marcet was the social worker who was in charge of my care as an inpatient. She and I deal on a different level now as I work with brain injury clients. Sue has taken the place of a very special person in my life, Dr. Rita Oliverio, who moved to New York. We have taken our own trips to the lighthouses and gone on crisis visits together. I often seek her advice when I get confused, and I know she understands .

I still make mistakes with my friends and have to work harder to build meaningful relationships. But I have plenty of help and plenty of time.

I have made a resolution to survive this tidal wave that hit my family and friends. I believe more than ever today, in the power of hugs, the strength of loving, and the value of friendships.

We all must be proud of the beauty within ourselves. We have the force of the oceans within us, a force that can carry us anywhere we dare to dream we can go. I know who I am and I am proud of where I'm finally going.

CHAPTER TWENTY-THREE

REVISITING THE BEACH

Oh, there are still days when I feel like one solitary seagull fighting against the world. But when that feeling engulfs me, I try to think of just soaring wherever the wind takes me. I know my direction in life has changed many times. I, also, know that my recovery has been meaningful, exciting and full of new experiences. It has made me who I am today. It has been a successful journey, because of its new learning, sudden changes, surprise beginnings, unexpected rewards and "never endings".

But I know too, the effect that brain injury has had on me, is just a part of the whole picture. Those around me, my husband, children, parents, friends, therapy teams, colleagues (and just about anyone who comes into contact with me), while I am continuing to grow and learn, have been and will change too, because of that injury. Perhaps it is even harder for them. They are the unsung heroes, but with help, proper information and support, they will be better equipped to deal with the overwhelming problems they face.

With education, hopefully that journey through brain injury, that once left everyone floundering in the wake of the tidal wave as it passed, will slowly turn into one of understanding. Brain injury of any kind affects not only the person who sustains it, but whoever touches them.

I know one thing very well. I am a very fortunate person. Most persons with brain injury do not get the excellent care, support and rehabilitation that I have received. Many persons get nothing, not even validation. What has happened to me, and how far along I am in "becoming", and in dealing and understanding my own injury, is directly related to that help, education and support. I have had the best family support, therapists and counselors all along the continuum of care. Maybe my rehabilitative process can be used as an example of what can be done, when people work together to provide the very best. I do not feel that I have to apologize for having had the best I could get. But I do feel sorry for others, who have trouble even getting into the support system.

Many people have asked me if I thought I would have recovered over time, to this extent, without formal rehabilitation. My answer is very simple. "No!" I believe that I would have been dead in less than two months after my second injury, from walking into the street and not knowing that I was unable to recognize danger and use good judgment.

Dead is forever. Only my specialized rehabilitation team discovered that glaring deficit and worked tirelessly to help me regain the ability to be safely independent. It took years, even with the best of help.

If I had somehow managed to stay alive over the past three years, would I have recovered? No one knows for sure. It would not have been as quickly and I would have been left with secondary scars that heal very slowly if ever. We have to make our own decisions on the course to take.

*If we always knew the answers,
there would be no growth from trying,
no lessons learned from doing,
and no feeling worse than dying
from the never-ending struggle
of clawing our way out.*

We need to join forces and learn from each other. Persons with brain injury working together can begin to empower themselves and become a conduit for advocacy for other survivors. Working with family and friends to understand the needs of all concerned, can help everyone involved find emotional, financial and physical support for each other.

If we can prevent only ONE person in our country from sustaining a brain injury, it would be worth all the education it takes and all the awareness we can provide.

For myself, I will continue to work with persons who have sustained brain injury and do whatever I can to make their lives easier. I am only one. But I am proud of who I am. We do move on with life, but the past doesn't go away. People ask me on occasion, why I don't leave the survivor label behind and get on with being "normal"(whatever that is). After all, no one recognizes me as having a problem.

But I feel an obligation to be who I am...to speak out for those who can't or won't...and to try to lead the way.

One of the hardest parts of recovering from a brain injury is that there are few heroes to emulate. As soon as people recover to the point of anonymity, most flee and try to resume their former lives, leaving other survivors struggling. We all need heroes. Every person who has sustained a brain injury is a hero....the real hero. Someone that they trust on their team needs to make sure they know that.

We need to always be aware of who we really are. Just when I think I have moved beyond a certain point, I run into that door of reminders, letting me know that my deficits are still there. Sometimes it is a heavy door to open....

TRANSITIONS

*When I wish that I could change
some things in me, I see.
Or be that other person,
That I know I used to be.
I know that it won't solve things
Or make me feel content.
To know that what I once was
Had just got up and went.*

*I plan to do so many things
I never did and more,
That each day brings new challenges,
I never faced before.
So I am working hard to learn
And have faith that it's okay,
To trust and place my future in
The "me" I am today.*

I have learned now to float with the tide. So each time that door shuts now reminding me of any limitations, I run quickly to open a window.

As that window rises, sometimes it is the sound of music that I hear, or the salt air that I smell, or the feel of a breeze blowing over those wildflowers in the meadow. Sometimes it is the sight of that angel left in the snow or sand. Whatever reminder it is, I am happy. I know that I was a part of making it. That makes me feel proud of who I am and how far I have come.

No one knows if, or when, the journey will end. No one even knows where the journey will go. For journeys through brain injury are as uncertain today as the weather in Maine and as vast as the oceans.

But I realize now, how much I am like that ocean. I have my lows and highs. Sometimes I rage out of control, yet I have an inner peace that lies just under the surface. Sometimes it is the other way around. The desire comes from within myself. I have the strength of self-renewal and the courage to try to take control of my life again. I have the inner power to cleanse, refresh, awaken and arouse. I have always had the desire to sing, the need to dance and the will to dream.

I believe in the sanctity of miracles, and the power in becoming...but never reaching. It is that oceanic struggle within, that makes us all go on.

Like the sea, I am ever-changing. In the process of my meandering, hopefully I will touch others as I move across the sands and they, in turn will touch me. And though we cannot always find the answers during our journey, we are ever searching and struggling to understand what the problems really are.

If all goes naturally, our answers will be found somewhere in the middle, along the coastline. It is here, where the ocean meets the shore...where movement meets stillness, where flowing liquid meets solid mass, where brute force meets tiny pebbles, where possibility meets reality, where the roaring waves meet their match at the end of the line...where we can sit or stand and watch the two separate forces, giving and taking, attacking and retreating. Sound familiar?

It is a two-way process, a mutuality that lets the shore take all the beating that the ocean can muster at high tide, and yet display its own majestic beauty in the sand and rocks as the water moves back and gives them room to "be".

When we meet at that coastline, we each become that solitary seagull, taking from the ocean one perspective, and giving back a beauty that enriches us all.

No one has the answers to life's problems, or the answers to surviving brain injury in an unforgiving world. But we all have the power within us to love and care for each other, to search for solutions, to help educate, to comfort those who grieve, to be silent no more, and to never, ever give up.

Part of us, sometimes our problems, sometimes our hopes and dreams, will be carried to wherever oceans go. But we must make sure that we all do our best to be there to meet the next tide, the next wave, the next challenge that needs answers, or the next person who needs help.

We must be ready with the "buoylines" of education, the "liferings" of compassion, and safety vests of hope.

We must make sure that we all do our best to leave our angel imprint waiting...............

SOLITARY SEAGULL

Sometimes, alone I watch the tide
And wonder where it goes.
I watch the waves coming rolling in
And settle around my toes.

The icy foam surrounds my feet
As I sink in grains of sand,
Renewing me...refreshing me
When the world gets out of hand.

The wind, the waves the rounded rocks
The smell of salted air,
Are things that refresh my soul
When nothing else is there.

The times I stand and watch the sea
Are times that I hold close.
That special port, my last resort,
For when I need it most.

When my world seems out of reach,
I reclaim the place I know.
Patiently, standing watch
As high tide turns to low.

The receding tide draws me in
Renews my strength of mind.
Together, we head outward
And leave the land behind.

One old solitary seagull,
Heading homeward, soaring low,
Taking all my worries with it
To wherever oceans go.

CHAPTER TWENTY-FOUR

EPILOGUE:

THE CALL OF THE GULLS

I have no more quarters stored in the tray between the seats now. I must have passed the last toll booth on my journey. My car moves quietly and effortlessly down the darkened turnpike. I told Gordon that I would be home before the Monday night football started on television at 9, and I know he'll begin to worry.

As I struggle to turn my body in such a way as to be able to turn on the overhead lightswitch and check the time, my car swerves toward the side of the road. In the path of the headlights, I see the mile marker illuminated. Mile #30! Oh my God! I'm going South, not North.

I recognize the sign for Old Orchard Beach,

and I can hear the gulls in the distance, guffawing at my predicament. I need to make a very quick decision. Should I attempt an illegal U-turn to go back the same way I came, or exit at Saco to head homeward over the western foothills?

Do you think I will make the U-turn and take the shorter route? Don't be ridiculous. I've learned to make good judgments. Going northwest is more isolated, but much more beautiful at night with the moon roof open.

Hesitantly, as if frozen in time, I find myself laughing for no apparent reason, as I reach up and push the button that rolls back the auto skylight. The car and I are suddenly alive with the light of the moon and the twinkling of a million stars. The urge to grab them all excites me, but the incoming rush of cold, ocean air rustles my work papers, piled loosely on the empty seat beside me.

With the moonroof open, I think I hear a seagull, somewhere in the distance, and there is a part of me who wants to follow its flight. It is odd how one solitary seagull can change your focus completely.

I should find a phone and call Gordon to let him know I'll be late. He won't mind. After all, I'm not lost. I'll simply say I decided at the last minute to take the scenic route. He'll smile.

When I get home, I may even tell him, I was

taking the time leave this imprint for others to follow, my kind of "angel in the snow". He'll just shake his head, lean over and kiss me on the cheek, then wrap his arm around me as he carries my bag up the driveway.

I really love him a lot. We're making it together. No one ever promised that life would be easy.

The storm of brain injury may not be completely over, but our beach wall is strong and intact. We have learned the value in taking preventive measures, and building good foundations as the weather has always been unpredictable in Maine. We never know what the future holds. But our roads are clear and our cellar is dry.

I know now that we are all part of that tidal wave...storm.. beachcomber ... driftwood... gull... ocean...   We are all stronger because of the storm.

Finding the determination to set new destinations in my writing goals, discovering the excitement of new ports of call in my work challenges, and returning home to a supportive family and friends encouraging me to leave the safety of the harbor, have made me who I am. They are the necessities of my survivorship.

I do go slower now, taking one day at a time. I thank God each morning I awaken, and try to pack as much love and laughter into each day as if it were my last. Someday I'll be right. Until then, well, we can only try to carve that legacy and leave an imprint...a kind of map for others to follow and believe in.

OH oh!...I can't forget the milk and bread I need to pick up. I wonder if I should get sour-dough or whole wheat, skim or low-fat. I think I'll wait until I find a store to decide. They may have only one kind and I may not even have to make a decision.

Now let's see. Should I take route 5 west or route 117 north? Decisions! No, they're merely challenges.

Anybody have a map?

Acknowledgments

I want to especially thank all of the people who encouraged me to write this book. It has been the hardest thing I have done since my injury.

To my children and husband, who shared their deepest feelings about our relationship, I love you more than ever. You are my strength and support.

To my friends who contributed their feelings and to those who couldn't, you are my inspiration.

To my team who worked with me, you are the hope for others who will follow me through brain injury recovery.

To all the other persons who sustain brain injury, remember tomorrow can be better.

To all the readers who finish this book, I hope you can follow the journey back and forth between events and friends and family. In real life, one affects the other and they are often, hard to separate. There are errors in the technical area of Oceans, but I offer no apologies. They are my badge of achievement.

I did it.

ORDERS:

Price per book $15.00
Add 6% sales tax in Maine

Add $1.75 Shipping & Handling 1st Book
$1.00 Each Additional

Make Check Payable to: Wings Publishing

MAIL OR FAX ORDER TO:
Wings Publishing
1 Clifford Court
So. Paris, Me. 04281
TEL & FAX # 207-743-8173

The following names are registered trademarks and I wish to acknowledge their importance and presence in the book.
I.B.M. International Business Machines
Aldus Pagemaker
WordPerfect
Nintendo Dr. Mario